IT'S NOT IF, IT'S WHEN:

What You Need to Know, Decide, and Share
Before the End-of-Life

A Practical Guide

by

Lynn Fitzgerald Macksey

ISBN 979-8-9954710-0-4 (Hardback)
ISBN 979-8-9954710-1-1 (Paperback)
ISBN 979-8-9954710-2-8 (eBook)

Published by LFM Enterprises, Inc.
Holly Springs, NC 27540-4001
www.alwayswithyou.com

Cover art courtesy of Pixabay user "pixifant" (https://pixabay.com/users/pixifant-2995268/, accessed February 2026)

Dedicated to:

My mother.

Acknowledgements

I am deeply grateful to the many colleagues and professionals who lent their time, expertise, and thoughtful attention to this project. Their insights strengthened this work in ways I would not have achieved alone.

My sincere thanks to **Sandra Sullivan**, MSN, ARNP-C, CVNP-C, and **Karen Cammarata**, RN, MSN, FNPC, whose careful reviews and substantive contributions helped refine both the clarity and clinical accuracy of these pages.

To **Tammy F. Trulock**, RN, thank you for your thoughtful review and for highlighting the sections that resonated most strongly. Your perspective helped me see the manuscript through the eyes of the bedside nurse I once was.

I am grateful to **Julie Lowery**, MS, CRNA, for her review of medical terminology and references. Your precision ensured that the language reflects both accuracy and respect for the disciplines represented here.

My appreciation also extends to **Phyllis Overton**, LPN, **Deborah Smith**, **Kevin Fitzgerald**, and **Kathy Miller**, RN, each of whom offered valuable review and feedback. Your willingness to read, reflect, and respond made this a stronger and more accessible resource for patients and families.

A special note of gratitude goes to friend and author **Jeanne Kalogridis** (aka J.M. Dillard), my primary editor. Her professional expertise, keen eye, and generous spirit guided this manuscript through its most important refinements. Jeanne's thoughtful edits—tightening language, smoothing tense shifts, and untangling more than a few comma splices—helped the work find its true voice. I am deeply appreciative of her thoroughness, her responsiveness, and the care she brought to every page.

To each of you: thank you for standing with me in this effort. Your contributions helped shape a book I hope will bring clarity, comfort, and confidence to those who need it most.

Contents

Introduction:

My Hopes For The Reader

As I write this book about death and dying, my hope is that it helps the reader feel less alone when confronting a subject most people quietly fear. I am not aiming to offer comfort through sentiment, but clarity through understanding. When people know what to expect — medically, emotionally, and practically — they can approach the end of life with steadier hands and clearer minds.

May this information help readers see that preparation is not morbid; it is responsible, compassionate, and deeply protective for the people they love. By thinking ahead, identifying priorities, and organizing what matters, they can face their fears and discover what is truly important to them, while sparing their family confusion, conflict, and the painful burden of guessing.

May this book also give readers language for conversations they have long avoided. Talking about death does not hasten it; silence only complicates it. Honest discussion opens the way to peace, dignity, and choices that reflect a person's true values.

For decades, I have wanted to write this book. I want to show how and why healthcare workers, nurses, physicians, and so many others do the work we do — whether we are helping someone recover or helping someone move toward a peaceful death.

While this book goes into detail about the choice of comfort care, I know there are people who want everything done… they want to stay alive, no matter what. And if that is your choice, I fully support it. You need to — and get to — choose the life, and the death, you want. Preparing for that death, and letting people know your wishes, is just as important as it is for someone who would choose comfort care.

Above all, I wish this book helps readers understand that preparing for death is an act of love — one that brings clarity to the living and peace to the dying.

Foreword

I have been a critical care nurse for forty-seven years, and on nearly every one of those days I have sat with families who had little understanding of what we do, why we do it, or how our interventions affect their hospitalized or critically ill loved ones. Calling this a frustrating problem — for me and for countless other healthcare workers — barely captures the depth of the issue.

This is one of the quiet, grinding realities of healthcare. Families are suddenly thrust into circumstances that require medical literacy, emotional readiness, and decision-making skills involving complex situations they've never had to navigate. Encountering this for the first time is like being dropped into a foreign country without a map. Many families simply haven't had the chance to develop the skills needed to make healthcare and end-of-life decisions.

Advance directive paperwork guidelines have helped people complete the forms, but has done far less to help them understand what those documents actually mean — or don't mean. What a person wants at the end of life, and what they absolutely do not want, is rarely as clear to patients or families as it should be.

Here is something most people don't realize: even if a patient has a living will in their chart, a single family member can tell the physician to "do everything," and everything will be done, regardless of what the patient wrote or discussed with their doctor. This is one of the most painful practical truths in end-of-life care. It is not universally true, but it is true often enough that clinicians talk about it as if it were. Why does this happen? Later in this book, you will learn how these conflicts arise and the practical steps families and clinicians can take to resolve them.

After working for three years as a critical care LPN, I attended the University of Florida's Bachelor of Nursing program, where I was required to write a senior thesis. I chose to focus on death and dying — specifically the issues of self-determination and living wills. Even then, I recognized how essential it is for people to understand their own health and the implications of their choices. Too often I found myself resuscitating a ninety-year-old patient who had arrived in our unit from a nursing home, while asking myself, and their attending physicians, "What's the goal?"

Over the years, I also worked in hospice, caring for patients and families at the end of life. That second job became a refuge from the futile, painful treatments we often delivered in the ICU to patients we could no longer help or heal. It was a break from hearing families insist, "God must decide," even when the patient was suffering.

Most of us move through life with a quiet assumption that death is something to think about "later." We postpone the conversation not because we are unwilling to face reality, but because we don't know where to begin. Preparation brings a quiet steadiness that comes from knowing nothing essential has been left unsaid or undone. It allows a person to shape the end of their life rather than being swept along by medical momentum or family anxiety.

Rather than offering an abstract philosophy, this book provides a steady, practical guide to help you reflect on what matters, speak openly, prepare thoughtfully, and live with purpose. Talking about death matters because silence leaves people unprepared. When the subject is avoided, decisions are made in crisis, values are guessed at, and families are forced to interpret what someone "would have wanted" at the very moment they are least able to think clearly. A single conversation held months or years earlier can spare loved one's confusion, conflict, and regret.

Discussing death also restores a sense of control. Naming what matters — comfort, dignity, independence, family presence, spiritual needs, medical limits — allows a person to shape the final chapter of their life rather than being carried along by events. It turns vague fears into concrete choices and replaces anxiety with clarity.

These conversations strengthen relationships. When people speak honestly about their hopes, fears, and priorities, they often discover a deeper understanding of one another. Families who talk openly about death tend to experience less guilt, less second-guessing, and more peace when the time comes.

Ultimately, talking about death while a person can still communicate their thoughts and wishes becomes an act of kindness — one that is deeply beneficial. It is a gift for the people who will one day stand at your bedside or settle your affairs. It says: "I have thought about this. I want to make this easier for you. Here is what matters to me." Waiting until the person grows too weak to articulate what they want is too late.

Preparation around death creates clarity because it replaces uncertainty with intention. When someone takes the time to articulate their values — comfort, dignity, independence, spiritual needs — medical limits and vague fears shift into practical guidance. Decisions that might otherwise fall to overwhelmed family members become clear instructions rooted in the person's own priorities. Guesswork disappears. Conflict fades. Loved ones follow a plan.

My purpose in offering this information is to help people understand how hospitals and all healthcare professionals view the complexities of medical care — and to show how informed, thoughtful preparation allows a person to face the end of life directly and with confidence.

PART I — TURNING TOWARD MORTALITY

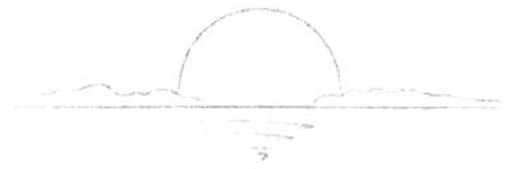

How can so many people be unprepared for one of life's near certainties?
— Jonathan Rauch

Chapter 1:

What is life in the context of death; and more importantly, a death with dignity?

It's a profound question. Talking about life in the context of death with dignity is essential because dignity at the end of life is deeply tied to how we understand what makes life meaningful.

1. Affirming the Value of Life First

Conversations about a dignified death begin with acknowledging what makes life meaningful in the first place. By naming what gives life value — relationships, autonomy, creativity, joy — we set the framework for what should be preserved or respected, even as life ends. These are the things people hold most dear.

2. Defining Quality of Life

Talking about life helps us ask: What makes life worth living for this person?
This shifts the focus from "How long can we prolong life?" to "What kind of life do we want to preserve?"

3. Continuity Between Living and Dying

Dying is not separate from life; it is the final chapter of living. By talking about life's meaning, we can see death with dignity not only as an ending, but as the culmination of how someone has lived.

4. Respecting Autonomy and Identity

Each person defines their life through their values, choices, and hopes. Discussing life makes it clear that end-of-life decisions should honor the same autonomy and identity that shaped the person's living years.

5. Highlighting Human Dignity

Dignity in dying is about preserving the dignity someone had in life. If life has been lived with respect, compassion, and agency, then death should reflect those same qualities.

6. Shaping Legacy and Memory

Conversations about life remind us that what endures is not just the fact of death, but the story of how a person lived. A dignified death allows loved ones to remember the fullness of the life lived, not only the struggle at the end.

Chapter 2:

What is death, and how has dying changed in the last century in the U.S.?

Definition of Death

It may sound surprising, but until the 1960s there was no legal definition of death in the United States because it was considered too obvious to require one. As medical technology advanced and made it possible to sustain functions that once would have ceased naturally, a formal definition became necessary. In 1963, Black's Law Dictionary offered this description: the cessation of life; the ceasing to exist; defined by physicians as a total stoppage of the circulation of the blood, and a cessation of the animal and vital functions consequent thereon, such as respiration and pulsation.

Death and Dying in the U.S. Before the 1950s

For most of human history, medicine has had limited ability to prevent illness, cure disease, or extend life. Reaching old age was often a matter of chance. In the United States before the 1950s, people with terminal illnesses were usually cared for at home and died surrounded by family. Because death occurred within the household, relatives were directly involved in caregiving and confronted the realities of dying firsthand. Much like birth, dying was primarily a family, community, and religious experience — not a medical one.

Death and Dying in the U.S. After the 1950s

In the mid-twentieth century, the longstanding tradition of dying at home shifted toward an institutional, technology-driven process. As hospitals expanded and medical technology advanced — ventilators, dialysis, intensive care units (ICUs) — clinicians could treat acute illness more aggressively and intervene immediately when a patient's condition worsened. Specialized staff, broader treatment options, and improved infection control made hospitals the default setting for serious illness and, increasingly, for death.

While these developments brought clear benefits, they also created a growing distance between the final stage of life and everyday living. The mobility of American society often separates younger and older generations, leaving many adults, even well into middle age, without firsthand experience caring for someone who is dying. A phone call announcing the death of a grandparent often replaces the intimate, communal experience that once accompanied the end of life. For many people, the most familiar images of dying now come from news and entertainment media, which tend to emphasize the sensational, the violent, or the sentimental — and rarely portray death as a social or relational event.

As medical capabilities expanded, societal expectations shifted as well. Death increasingly came to be viewed as a medical event to be managed and controlled in a hospital rather than a natural process supported at home. Changes in household structure and the rise of women working outside the home meant fewer family members were available to provide end-of-life care. Hospitals became the preferred, and often only, setting for dying, as the focus moved from comfort to attempts to prolong life through sophisticated interventions. Within this framework, death itself began to be seen as a kind of medical failure.

Americans today live far longer than they did at the end of the nineteenth century, and infant death — once common — has become rare, though disparities persist due to factors such as access to healthcare, prematurity, low birthweight, and poverty. The causes of death in old age now differ markedly from those that once claimed younger lives, and the typical experience of dying has changed just as dramatically. The result is a modern landscape in which death is both more distant from daily life and more medicalized than at any point in American history.

A Global Perspective

Dying in hospitals is not unique to the United States. In most high-income countries, deaths have shifted from the home to hospitals or other institutions over the past 70–80 years. But the pattern varies widely depending on culture and healthcare system structure. Middle-income countries show a mixed pattern, with urban hospital deaths and rural home deaths. In low-income countries, home deaths remain the norm because hospitals are scarce, transportation is limited, and cultural norms favor dying at home.

Chapter 3:

Everybody dies — why don't we talk about it?

The reality of death is unavoidable… it comes for everyone. It's never a question of if, only when. Yet despite this certainty, many people avoid talking about their own mortality. Why is it so difficult to speak — or even think — about our eventual death? We live in a world saturated with reminders of it. News outlets report deaths constantly, often highlighting the most tragic or sensational stories. Even when the media strives to balance public interest with compassion for grieving families, death is still presented in ways that feel distant or impersonal.

Talking about death is complicated because it touches every layer of human experience: cultural norms, social expectations, spiritual beliefs, emotional reactions, and cognitive defenses. Our reluctance is rooted in psychological, social, and spiritual factors. People fear the unknown, the loss of control, the possibility of suffering, or the pain of leaving loved ones behind. For many, the topic stirs sadness, regret, or reminders of unfinished business. Religious beliefs can also intensify anxiety, especially when tied to concerns about judgment or uncertainty about the afterlife.

In the United States, a culture of denial surrounds death. Intellectually, we know we will all die, but the topic is often pushed aside because it feels uncomfortable. This avoidance is not uniquely American, but it is particularly pronounced in our society, where death is minimized, sanitized, or kept at a distance. Denial may protect people from discomfort in the short term, but it can also be harmful, depriving families of meaningful moments at the end of life.

In American culture, death is frequently treated as an interruption rather than an inevitability. It conflicts with deeply held values such as optimism, productivity, and youthfulness, making it something to resist or ignore. This relentless positivity makes it hard for people to say, "I'm dying," "I'm exhausted," or "I want comfort instead of more treatment." The cultural script leaves little room for realism, grief, or acceptance. Youth is idealized, and aging is something to conceal or fight against. As a result, avoidance shapes how Americans age, how they seek medical care, and how they prepare — or fail to prepare — for the end of life.

In the United States, death and dying remain unpopular topics. Conversations about mortality are often dismissed as "morbid," and many people try to avoid them for as long as possible — just as they try to avoid death itself. Yet as Benjamin Franklin famously noted, "In this world, nothing is certain except death and taxes."

Death is also often viewed as a failure of the medical system rather than a natural part of life. This mindset fuels aggressive medical interventions even when death is near. In earlier generations, death commonly occurred at home and was woven into daily life. Today, most Americans die in hospitals or nursing homes, which shifts the dying process into institutional settings and distances it from families and communities. Many people have little direct experience with death until it touches them personally. With few everyday depictions of dying or death rituals, the subject becomes abstract and remote. This cultural distancing leaves many emotionally unprepared for loss.

Elizabeth Kübler-Ross once observed that denying death leads people to live "empty, purposeless lives," postponing what matters under the illusion of endless tomorrows. Her reminder is clear: the real concern is not the end of the physical body, but whether we truly live while we are alive.

Given all these fears and hesitations, what helps people come to terms with this fundamental reality of life?

Chapter 4:

Step 1: how we break through denial and name the reality

Usually, we do not begin thinking seriously about death and dying until something significant interrupts the rhythm of daily life and demands our attention. It might be having children, receiving a medical diagnosis, experiencing a loss or a close call, or simply noticing that we — or the people we love — are getting older. When mortality becomes real instead of theoretical, many of us find ourselves feeling anxious and unsure.

But waiting for a crisis leaves little room for clarity. The first step in preparing for your own death is far simpler and far less dramatic: acknowledging, plainly and without panic, that your life will one day end. This acknowledgment is not an emotional event; it is a practical one. It is the same kind of recognition we bring to other certainties in life — planning for retirement, maintaining our health, or caring for the people who depend on us. Naming the reality of death allows you to make decisions with intention rather than avoidance.

You do not need to have answers yet. You do not need to know what you want, how you feel, or what comes next. This chapter is about creating the mental space to think. It is about shifting from "I'll deal with that someday" to "This deserves my attention now." Once that shift happens, everything else becomes easier — the conversations, the planning, and even the emotional work that may follow.

Acknowledging mortality is not about dwelling on the end. It is about clearing the fog so you can see your life more clearly. Accepting the reality of your own death sharpens your focus, turning the thought into a mirror for your life's purpose. It is the foundation on which every other step in this book rests.

Gentle ways to begin thinking about your own mortality

Talking about death in general terms — or about someone else's death — can feel easier.

Know first that denial is normal. Denial isn't a flaw; it's a protective reflex. But denial thrives in silence.

Name the discomfort. Saying "I don't like thinking about death" is already a step toward clarity. Denial weakens when you put words to what you've been avoiding. Start with small, non-threatening reflections. Think about aging, change, or the passage of time — topics that sit adjacent to mortality but feel less overwhelming.

Keep focusing on what is useful, not frightening.

-- "What matters most to me in my final years?"

-- "What do I want my family to know?"

-- "What unfinished tasks would bring me peace if completed?"

Learn just enough to feel informed, not overwhelmed.

-- "What happens in a hospital at the end of life?"

-- "What documents do I need — and what do they actually do?"

-- "What does comfort-focused care look like?"

Use concrete, practical tasks as an entry point — the things you "should have done a long time ago," but can begin now. These tasks are not emotional confrontations; they are acts of responsibility. Yet they quietly open the door to thinking about death in a grounded way.

- Writing a Last Will and Testament

- Choosing a Durable Power of Attorney (DPOA) for healthcare

- Choosing a DPOA for financial matters

- Organizing important personal documents

Read or listen to people who speak about death with clarity. Memoirs, essays, films, or interviews where people reflect on dying can normalize the topic. Hearing others speak plainly about death helps you internalize that it is not a taboo subject. The documentary *How to Die in Oregon* is especially powerful.

Talk about it in low-stakes settings. Casual conversations with trusted people about aging parents, medical decisions, or cultural attitudes can make the topic feel less charged. You don't need to start with your own death; you can ease into it.

Reflect on what gives your life meaning. Thinking about your values, your priorities, and what you want people to remember about you naturally leads to a healthier acceptance of mortality. It's not morbid — it's clarifying. It helps you live with intention.

The goal is not to defeat denial but to make room for a fuller, calmer understanding of your own life. Healthy thinking about death isn't about dwelling on it; it's about removing the fear that keeps you from acknowledging it.

A simple but powerful exercise

Imagine you have one year left to live. Then one month. Then one week.

Ask yourself:

-- What becomes important?

-- What falls away?

This reframes mortality as a lens for clarity, not panic.

Part II — WHAT CHANGES WHEN YOU ACCEPT YOUR MORTALITY

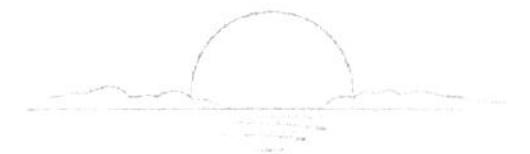

Life and death are one thread; the same line viewed from different sides.
— Lao Tzu

Chapter 5:

Acknowledging that your time is finite sharpens your priorities

Accepting your mortality does not shorten your life, darken your days, or diminish your hope. In fact, the opposite is often true. When people stop avoiding the reality of death, they frequently find that life becomes more focused, more intentional, and more aligned with what genuinely matters. This chapter explores how that shift happens and what it can mean for the way you live each day.

Decisions that once felt complicated become simpler. Obligations that never fit your values fall away. You begin to invest more energy in the relationships, routines, and commitments that reflect who you are, rather than who you think you are supposed to be. This clarity is steady, not dramatic. It allows you to move through life with a sense of direction rather than drift.

You may also notice changes in how you spend your time. You become more deliberate about what you say "yes" to and what you decline. You may find yourself more patient in some areas, less tolerant in others, and more aware of the moments that deserve your attention. Accepting mortality often brings a quiet discipline: a desire to use your days well — not by doing more, but by choosing more wisely.

Later chapters will show how preparation for death can lead to a more grounded, meaningful approach to living — one that reflects your values, honors your relationships, and gives you a sense of steadiness as you move forward.

You can sustain a grounded perspective when you integrate the reality of death in a way that steadies your life rather than disrupts it — because accepting mortality isn't a single moment of insight; it's a practice.

Chapter 6:

Understanding your values

Before you can make meaningful decisions about the end of your life, you need to understand what truly matters to you. Not what you think *should* matter, not what others *expect* to matter, but the handful of principles, priorities, and relationships that *genuinely shape the way you want to live* — and the way you hope to be remembered.

Most people have never taken the time to name these values directly. They show up in habits, preferences, and reactions, but rarely in clear language. This chapter helps you identify those underlying priorities so that every choice you make — from medical decisions to personal messages to practical planning — reflects who you are rather than who circumstances push you to be.

When your life gets quiet and the noise stops, what rises to the surface? Fear, hope, relationships, regret? Your mind gravitates toward what matters, even when you're not trying.

Reflection

- *Pay attention to what drains your energy versus what steadies you. This is one of the clearest indicators of values. What gives you a sense of purpose, calm, or satisfaction? What leaves you feeling depleted or angry?*

- *Look at how you spend your time — where your energy goes, what you protect, the things you make room for even on busy days.*

- *Ask yourself, if everything else fell away, what would I want preserved? Which relationships? Which routines or rituals? If you had to choose only a few things to carry forward, those are your priorities.*

- *Reflect on moments in your life when you felt most like yourself. What were you doing? Who were you with? What values were being honored?*

Notice what you defend — your family, independence, integrity, time, health, peace. What you guard reveals what you value.

Understanding your values is not a philosophical exercise. It is a practical tool. When you know what you stand for, decisions become simpler. Conflicts become easier to navigate. Conversations with loved ones become clearer. And the plans you put in place feel less like paperwork and more like a continuation of your life's intentions.

You do not need perfect clarity to begin. You only need curiosity and honesty. As you work through this chapter, you will start to see patterns: what gives your life meaning, what you want to protect, what you are willing to let go of, and what you hope others will understand about you when you are no longer here to explain it.

One last question: "*What would I want people to know about me if I couldn't speak for myself?*"

- What I believe.

- What I hope for.

- What I fear.

- What I absolutely do not want.

- What I want my life to reflect.

These questions cut through the noise quickly and are especially important in the context of end-of-life preparation.

Your values are the compass for everything that follows. Before you talk with anyone, before you sign anything, before you make a single plan, you deserve to know what direction you want to face. Values can shift as life changes, so revisit these questions as circumstances evolve.

Author's note – perfection vs. excellence

Recently, I came across a story by writer Nicole Johnson about her grandmother's lifelong pursuit of perfection, and it stopped me in my tracks. Her grandmother had built her world around strict order and the belief that flawless effort was both possible and necessary. Nicole grew up determined to be different, imagining a home where kids could be messy, spontaneous, and free. But once she became a mother herself, she found that same urge to control creeping into her own life, tightening around her days until everything felt like a test she had to pass. The pressure of raising four children while trying to maintain an idealized version of family life left her exhausted and trapped in a loop she couldn't break.

Then her grandmother fell ill, and the illusion of perfection suddenly looked small compared to the reality of limited time. As her health declined, she began letting go of the little things — matching accessories, spotless rooms, constant self-monitoring. She started asking for help. Her new mantra, "Don't sweat it," became a kind of permission slip to live differently.

Watching her grandmother release decades of impossible expectations helped Nicole do the same. She realized she didn't need to wait until old age or illness to loosen her grip. When her grandmother saw how hard she was pushing herself, she told her plainly that perfection was an illusion, not a goal. Then she asked the question that shifted everything: *Did you do your best?* That simple reframing changed the way Nicole approached her life.

Her story stayed with me. I've always liked to think I'm steering the ship of my life — that if I work hard enough, I can make everything turn out the way I want. But the more I pushed myself toward perfection, the more anxious and unsettled I became. Nicole's story helped me see that she wasn't just describing her grandmother; she was describing a pattern many of us carry without noticing. It made me look more closely at the difference between perfection and excellence.

Perfection demands control. It is rigid, anxious, arrogant. It's delaying a task because the conditions aren't ideal. It's tucking behind the illusion that if we just try harder, we can avoid mistakes, disappointment, or vulnerability.

Excellence, by contrast, is grounded, humane, and sustainable. It asks only that we bring our full effort to the moment we're in — not that we control every outcome. Excellence leaves room for being human.

Chapter 7:

What you want your life to stand for

Once you begin to understand your values, the next step is to consider how those values shape the story of your life. Every person leaves a legacy, whether they intend to or not. It is not limited to grand achievements or public recognition. Legacy is the lasting mark your choices, relationships, and actions leave on the people who continue living after you're no longer here.

Thinking about legacy is not about crafting a perfect narrative. It is about identifying the themes that have guided you — your commitments, your priorities, your lessons learned — and deciding how you want those themes to be understood. When you take the time to articulate what your life stands for, you give others clarity. You also give yourself a sense of continuity: the reassurance that your life has coherence and direction, even as it nears its final chapters.

A large part of this book is meant to help you translate your values into a practical understanding of your legacy. You will reflect on the roles you have played, the relationships that have shaped you, and the principles that have guided your decisions. You will get to consider what you want others to remember, what you want to pass on, and what unfinished messages or intentions deserve attention now rather than later.

Legacy is not about perfection. It is about honesty. It is about choosing what you want to emphasize, what you want to clarify, and what you want to leave behind in a way that feels true to who you are.

Chapter 8:

What we leave behind – leaving a legacy

A legacy, in practical terms, is the lasting impact you create through your actions, values, and stories. It extends beyond your lifetime and becomes both a guide for the people living now and a gift to those who come after you. Legacy includes tangible things like property or keepsakes, but it also includes the intangible: wisdom, traditions, character, and the way you have lived your life. It is not about money alone. It is about shaping your life with intention now so that what you leave behind reflects purpose, meaning, and the connections you've built across generations.

Begin by reflecting on the difference you want to make and choosing to live intentionally.

Legacy acts as a compass, helping align daily choices with your core values and giving life a sense of purpose beyond yourself.

Tangible expressions of legacy may include:

- *Letters, photos, or recorded messages*

- *Flash drives with meaningful songs*

- *Favorite pictures of you with the people you love*

- *Property, keepsakes, and personal notes*

But legacy is also deeply internal. It is what you leave behind; and it's what you leave within people. The way you listened, the way you showed up, the way you handled hardship. These become part of the emotional DNA of the people who knew you.

Legacy lives in the stories families tell, the phrases they repeat, the small rituals they keep alive. Loved ones often value these most.

Vignette About legacy

A 29-year-old with a terminal brain tumor didn't fear death as much as being forgotten. He recorded short videos — not dramatic messages, just everyday moments: making coffee, talking about music, laughing at his own jokes. He said, "I want them to remember how I sounded when I was alive." His reckoning was about legacy, not in the grand sense, but in the deeply human one:

I was here. I mattered.

Chapter 9:

Working with regrets at the end of life

Thinking about death is uncomfortable and often a little frightening, so it's understandable that it rarely makes anyone's "to-do today" list. Yet it is part of life, and many people reach the end carrying regrets. Regret is not a moral failing; it's a signal — a pointer toward unfinished business, unspoken words, or priorities that deserve attention while there's still time. Regret is the recognition that something in the past still tugs at you. These regrets can be as small as turning down the sweet kid from math class who asked you to prom, or as life-shaping as not moving to Colorado at twenty-five. The encouraging truth is that even decades-old regrets can still be worked with in meaningful ways.

There are two broad categories of regret. **Regrets of commission** are the things we wish we *hadn't* done: saying hurtful things, ending a relationship harshly, lying when honesty mattered, compromising integrity for approval or convenience, making rash decisions in anger, letting pride block reconciliation, or pushing people away out of fear or self-doubt.

Regrets of omission are the things we wish we *had* done: expressing affection or gratitude, showing up for birthdays and milestones, having difficult conversations, apologizing, leaving a job that never fit, choosing courage over fear, or defending someone who needed support.

Common end-of-life regrets often sound like:

- I spent too much time worrying about being judged.

- I wish I had taken more risks.

- I wish I hadn't waited for the "right time" to live… like after retirement or after the kids were grown.

- I wish I had traveled more and experienced other cultures.

- I worked too much and missed what mattered.

- I wish I had expressed my feelings honestly, especially "I love you."

- I wish I had spoken up when something mattered.

- I wish I had nurtured my friendships instead of letting them fade.

- I wish I had taken better care of myself — even something as simple as flossing my teeth.

- I wish I had been more patient with my children.

- I wish I had been a better spouse.

- I wish I had let myself be happier.

- I wish I had forgiven myself and others instead of holding onto anger.

- I wish I had taken more pictures — of others and of myself — instead of hiding from the camera because I thought I looked "bad."

- I waited too long to accept and flow with life. I stressed over things I couldn't change.

- I wish I could have laughed at the chaos and confusion of life instead of making myself miserable trying to control it.

Regret becomes heavier when it stays vague. If there is a hurt that matters to you, name it — to yourself and, if possible, to the person involved. Many people feel relief simply by saying, "I wish I had…," "I'm sad that I didn't…," or "I regret how I handled…." Naming regret doesn't make it worse; it opens the door to healing.

If you cannot speak directly to the person you hurt, tell the truth to someone who can hold it — a family member, a friend, a chaplain, a trusted caregiver. Being witnessed can bring profound peace.

Some regrets will remain unresolved. Some relationships stay estranged. Some words are never spoken. Some choices cannot be undone. Even so, peace is still possible. Acknowledging the truth without trying to rewrite it is its own form of acceptance. No one is the sum of their worst moments. Reflect on what you learned, how you grew, how you loved, what you contributed, and who you became. This restores a sense of wholeness.

Regret is not a sign of failure; it is a sign of awareness. It can be surprisingly useful. Regret can motivate change, clarify what truly mattered, illuminate essential relationships, and help release old conflicts. It can open the door to conversations, apologies, forgiveness, and reconciliation. Acknowledging regret helps release guilt, accept our humanity, and make peace with the story of our life.

Regret is, in the end, a form of emotional housekeeping — a clearing space for peace.

Chapter 10:

Forgiving yourself for all the things you've spent years criticizing

Talking about regrets becomes much more powerful when self-forgiveness isn't treated as an optional addition but as the natural next step in the emotional arc. Once regret has clarified what matters, forgiveness becomes the work of releasing self-punishment so you can live those values more fully now. You can emphasize self-accountability without self-cruelty. Forgiving yourself doesn't erase responsibility for what you did — it allows you to carry it with clarity instead of self-attack.

I don't care who you are or what you do, everyone makes mistakes. Even the Dalai Lama has surely said things he wishes he hadn't. All of us carry moments we're not proud of, from the small missteps to the choices so painful we never speak of them. I certainly have mine. These are the things I've done that I regret deeply — the ones I've never admitted to anyone, not even to my closest friends.

I've had to learn how to forgive myself, because there is no going back to rewrite what happened. Some of the people I hurt are no longer alive. Others are people I no longer have in my life — and don't want in my life anymore. Self-forgiveness became the only path left, not because the past disappears, but because living in permanent self-punishment doesn't honor anyone, including the people I wronged.

So, if you wronged someone, you could seek their forgiveness, but it is even more important to offer forgiveness to yourself. "I did the best I could with who I was then. I forgive myself for being human." Self-forgiveness is not self-excusing; it is self-liberating.

Forgiveness

♥ *Let go. Live simply. Love generously. Speak truthfully.
Work diligently.*

♥ *Stop moving. Pause to appreciate your family, your
home, a hot shower, and the breath you are taking in
this moment.*

♥ *Love your life by trusting your intuition, taking chances,
losing and finding happiness, cherishing your memories,
and learning through experience. You might not end up
exactly where you intended to go, but you will eventually
arrive precisely where you need to be.*

Part III — CONVERSATIONS THAT MATTER

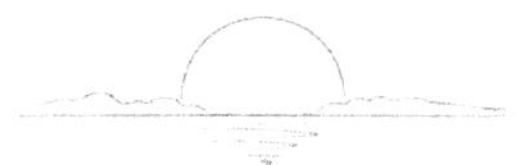

If we cannot speak of death, we cannot prepare for it.
— Unknown author

Your choices are your voice. If you don't speak them, others must guess.
— Contemporary advance-directive guidance

Planning for the end-of-life is not about dying. It's about how you want to live until the very last moment. — Palliative care principle

Talking about death won't make it happen, but not talking about it won't stop it.
— Common hospice teaching

Chapter 11:

Getting ready to talk about death with others

By the time you reach this chapter, you've already done the quiet internal work: acknowledging your mortality, identifying your values, and beginning to understand the story you want your life to tell. The next step is bringing these insights into the open so you can share them with the people who need to hear them. For many, this is the hardest part — not because the topic is complicated, but because it feels unfamiliar.

The most challenging part of talking about death is accepting our mortality: the reality that we, and the people we love, will eventually die. It is natural to feel afraid. Most of us don't know what to expect, and we don't know when it will happen. It's tempting to avoid the subject entirely and "cross that bridge when we get to it." But avoidance often deepens fear. What we refuse to face grows larger in the dark.

Death does not have to be viewed as a frightening event at the end of life. Talking about it allows us to see it as a natural part of living — something that can be approached with peace, clarity, and even purpose. These conversations also make the topic less intimidating for the next generation, especially children, who learn from our willingness to speak honestly.

Avoiding the subject doesn't prevent difficulty; it simply delays it. Open communication reduces confusion, prevents conflict, and gives everyone a shared understanding of what matters most. Communicating without sentimentality means using clear language, being honest, and focusing on presence rather than trying to "fix" emotions. This approach respects both the reality of the situation and the depth of the other person's feelings.

Since death is inevitable, developing coping skills becomes essential. Thinking about our own mortality — though uncomfortable at first — can be a powerful starting point. Reflecting on the reality of our final days helps clarify what truly matters and affirms our hopes for how we want to live, and ultimately, how we want to die. This kind of reflection highlights what is most important:

comfort, dignity, spiritual peace, being surrounded by loved ones, or ensuring that our medical wishes are respected. It also helps us release what matters less — unfinished projects, external expectations, or the pressure to "do it all" — and instead focus on what brings meaning. Sometimes this awareness even inspires us to live with greater purpose.

By acknowledging our mortality, we move from avoidance to intentionality. We gain the ability to prepare — emotionally, spiritually, and practically — for the end of life. This not only reduces anxiety but also allows us to live more fully in the present, making choices that align with our deepest values.

Coping often includes open conversations with family and friends. Sharing your thoughts and wishes creates opportunities for meaningful exchanges, such as telling a child, "I am so proud of you," or offering an overdue "I'm sorry." These conversations shift our focus toward living more consciously. Recognizing our mortality clarifies our values and strengthens our purpose. Support from spiritual leaders, journaling, or working with counselors, social workers, or chaplains can also help create space for acceptance.

Many people avoid talking about their own death with family because they fear upsetting loved ones or sparking conflict. Others feel unprepared or overwhelmed by the emotional weight of the conversation. Practical and legal preparations, like writing a will, are often postponed for the same reasons.

Most of us were never taught how to talk about death. We learn how to discuss careers, finances, and family plans, but not how to express our wishes for the end of life. As a result, even simple conversations can feel awkward or emotionally charged. This chapter is designed to remove that pressure. Talking about death does not require perfect timing, special language, or dramatic declarations. It requires clarity, steadiness, and a willingness to begin.

The next chapter concerns having conversations with the people who matter. It will help you choose the right moment, frame the conversation in a natural way, and speak plainly without alarming or overwhelming others. You will also learn how to navigate common reactions such as discomfort, avoidance, humor, or silence, which often arise when people are unsure how to respond.

The goal is not to have one perfect conversation. The goal is to open a door. Once the door is open, the rest becomes easier: sharing your wishes, asking questions, clarifying responsibilities, and ensuring that the people around you understand what matters most.

Talking about death is ultimately an act of care. It creates certainty where there might otherwise be confusion. It gives your loved ones guidance instead of guesswork. And it allows you to live with confidence that your intentions are known.

Language That Opens the Door

A gentle beginning often starts with simply reflecting on what matters most to you. The goal is not to deliver a speech — it's to create space. Door-opening language is honest, calm, and invitational.

Acknowledge the difficulty

"I feel a little scared, but I want us to have this conversation."

Invite connection

- "I've been thinking about what matters most to me, and I'd like to share some of it with you."

- "Can we talk about something important to me? It's not urgent — I just want you to know my wishes."

- "I want to make things easier for you someday, and that means being clear about what I want."

- "I've been reflecting on my values, and I'd like to talk about how they guide my decisions for the future."

- "This isn't about anything happening right now. It's just something I want us to understand together."

Language That Closes the Door

These phrases tend to trigger fear, defensiveness, or emotional shutdown:

- "We need to talk about what happens when I die."

- "You'll have to deal with this when I'm gone."

- "If something happens to me, you're on your own."

These phrases, when expressed, can create pressure instead of openness. A softer approach keeps the conversation human and manageable.

Finally, trying to express everything at once can leave your mind overwhelmed and frozen. Break the process into small, human-sized steps and the conversation becomes far more manageable.

Chapter 12:

How to have conversations with people who matter

Talking about death with family is different from talking about it with anyone else. Loved ones bring history, emotion, and their own fears into the room. They may worry about losing you, about making mistakes, or about saying the wrong thing. These reactions are not signs that the conversation should be avoided; they simply reflect how much the relationship matters. Your task is not to persuade or perform. Your task is to speak with steadiness, offer clarity, and invite your family into a process that unfolds over time.

These conversations are not really about death. They are about care, responsibility, and protecting the relationships that matter most.

Your role and theirs

When you talk with your family about your wishes, your role is simple: share what matters to you — your values, your priorities, and the kind of care you want if you cannot speak for yourself. You do not need to have every detail figured out. You only need to offer enough clarity that your loved ones won't be left guessing later.

Their role is equally straightforward: to listen, ask questions, and understand your wishes, even if the conversation feels emotional or unfamiliar. They are not expected to predict medical outcomes or agree on every detail. Their purpose is to represent your voice when you cannot.

These conversations may stir sadness, fear, or silence. That is normal. What everyone can expect, however, is a shared understanding of your priorities and less confusion in the future. Talking about your death is ultimately an act of care; it gives your loved ones guidance instead of uncertainty and allows you to live with confidence that your intentions are known.

Guiding principles for family conversations

- **Honesty is grounding.** Clear, direct language helps everyone breathe a little easier.

- **Do not minimize someone's pain.** Each person's reaction is shaped by their own history and fears.

- **Presence matters.** A quiet moment, a gentle touch, or steady eye contact often communicates more than long explanations.

- **Acknowledge emotion without trying to fix it.** "I can see how much this hurts" can be more supportive than any solution.

- **Sharing your wishes is not a burden.** It is kindness. You are not asking your family to carry your emotional weight — you are giving them the gift of clarity.

Start small

A first conversation does not need to cover everything. Begin with two simple topics:

- What feels important in your life right now?

- How do you feel about your own mortality?

Starting with the present keeps the conversation grounded in identity rather than fear. When people name what matters to them — relationships, routines, values — they reconnect with their sense of self. When they gently explore their feelings about death, they begin to understand what they hope for, what they fear, and what they want their loved ones to know. From there, the conversation can unfold naturally over time.

Choosing the right moment

There is no perfect time to talk about death, but some moments make the conversation easier. Look for times when both you and the other person are calm, unhurried, and able to focus. These conversations rarely go well when someone is stressed, exhausted, or already in crisis.

Often, the best openings arise naturally:

- after a medical appointment

- during a quiet evening at home

- while organizing paperwork

- when someone mentions aging, illness, or the loss of a friend

A good moment is one in which:

- you feel steady enough to speak clearly

- the other person is emotionally available

- there is enough time to talk without rushing privacy allows honesty

You don't need a dramatic setup — just a pause in the noise of daily life.

Keep the conversation small and manageable

- "I'd like to talk about one part of my wishes today."

- "Can we start with what matters most to me if I'm ever seriously ill?"

Begin with the present, not the end

Start by talking about what matters to you while you are living. What:

- brings comfort, joy, or peace

- relationships you want to protect

- responsibilities you hope will be handled with care

Then gently name your fears. Of:

- suffering

- losing autonomy

- burdening others

- being forgotten

Fears often reveal what someone values most. If you cannot articulate what you want, begin with what you *don't* want:

-- "I don't want to be kept alive if I can't recognize my family."

-- "I don't want aggressive interventions if they won't restore meaningful life."

-- "I don't want my loved ones to feel guilty."

Negatives create boundaries. Boundaries create clarity.

From there, move toward what you *do* want:

- preferred medical interventions

- comfort measures (shift in medical care; focus on symptom management)

- where you want to be

- who you want present

- what dignity means to you

This is where advanced directives and DPOA choices naturally emerge.

Finally, share your emotional legacy:

- messages of love

- apologies or reconciliations

- gratitude

- hopes for the people you leave behind

This is not about perfection. It is about authenticity.

Handling resistance, emotion, and silence

Resistance is usually fear in disguise. When someone says, "I don't want to talk about this," they are often expressing anxiety, not rejection.

Gentle responses keep the door open:

-- "I understand. We don't have to talk about everything today."

-- "I just want you to know my wishes, so things are easier for you someday."

-- "We can take this one step at a time."

Tears, frustration, or worry are normal. You don't need to fix emotions — just make space for them.

-- "I can see this is hard."

-- "It's okay to feel whatever you're feeling."

-- "We can pause if you need to."

Your steadiness helps others stay grounded. Silence is not a problem. It is processing. Allow the pause.

When tension rises, return to the purpose:

-- "I'm bringing this up because I care about you."

-- "I want to make things easier for everyone later."

-- "This is about clarity, not crisis."

If, after several attempts, your loved ones simply cannot or will not engage, consider recording a video message:
-- "This is how I feel."
-- "This is what I want."
-- "This is what matters to me."
It may feel less threatening to them and still opens the door.

Separating wants, needs, and non-negotiables

When people talk about end-of-life wishes, everything tends to get lumped together — hopes, fears, preferences, and absolute boundaries. Sorting these into **wants**, **needs**, and **non-negotiables** brings order to a topic that often feels overwhelming. It also gives families and healthcare teams a clearer roadmap when decisions must be made quickly.

Wants

Things that would make the end of life better, but are not essential:

- certain foods

- music

- rituals or routines

Needs

Elements that must be in place for you to feel safe, respected, and cared for:

- adequate pain and symptom control

- emotional or spiritual support

- clear communication from the medical team

- a calm environment

- respect for cultural or religious practices

- the presence (or absence) of certain people

Non-negotiables - Boundaries that must be honored:

- "I do not want to be kept alive on a ventilator."

- "I do not want CPR if my heart stops."

- "I do not want feeding tubes."

- "I want comfort-focused care only."

- "I do not want to die in a hospital."

- "I want my healthcare proxy, not my entire family, making decisions."

Simple exercise to clarify your own list

- *Write three columns: Wants, Needs, Non-negotiables.*

- *Fill them in without overthinking.*

- *Revisit the list a few days later and refine it.*

- *Share it with the person who will speak for you if you cannot speak for yourself.*

- *Update it every year or after major life changes.*

This is not about predicting the future — it is about giving your loved ones clarity instead of uncertainty.

Why these distinctions matter

For families:

They prevent conflict by clarifying what is optional, what is essential, and what is absolutely off-limits.

For clinicians:

They provide a clear, actionable framework that aligns treatment with your values.

For you, they:

- transform fear into intention.

- turn vague hopes into practical guidance.

- ensure your voice is heard even when you cannot speak.

When family members disagree

Disagreement does not mean the conversation has failed. It often means people care in different ways. The most effective approach is to return everyone to the same foundation: **your values and what you have clearly stated matters to you.**

Remind them:

- the goal is not to win an argument

- the goal is to honor your choices

If emotions rise, slow the conversation down, restate your intentions, and focus on areas of agreement. Reassure your family that you are not asking them to solve everything today — you are giving them guidance, so they won't have to struggle later.

Why these conversations matter

When loved ones are uncertain about your wishes, it can add turmoil to an already painful time. Lack of planning creates anxiety, conflict, and unnecessary guilt.

Think of it this way: if two family members disagreed about who should receive a cherished item, wouldn't you want to be there to understand their feelings and resolve it fairly? Honest conversations now help protect relationships later.

Talking about death is also a way to deepen meaning. As Elizabeth Kübler-Ross observed, recognizing that we all share the same fate can help us appreciate both our differences and our shared humanity. Awareness of mortality often prompts people to reflect more intentionally on their goals and to choose what truly supports their well-being.

When we understand that death is not a personal failure but a universal truth, the conversation becomes less threatening. It becomes a way to live more intentionally, clarify what matters, and protect the people we love from confusion and conflict later.

Emotional and relational preparation

As you consider the end of your life, you may notice relationships you want to strengthen, conversations you want to finish, and small but meaningful pieces of unfinished business you want to address. This chapter focuses on those human details — the ones that never appear on legal forms but matter deeply to the people you love.

Emotional preparation is not about fixing every feeling or repairing every relationship. It is not an attempt to rewrite the past. Instead, it is about recognizing what deserves attention while you still have the time and clarity to act.

For some, this may mean expressing gratitude or appreciation. For others, it may involve clearing up a misunderstanding, offering reassurance, acknowledging the importance of a relationship, or apologizing for past hurt.

These gestures do not need to be dramatic. Small, sincere efforts often carry the greatest weight. They clarify what matters, soften old tensions, and reduce the chance of future regret.

You can also consider the kind of support your loved ones may need — practical, emotional, or otherwise — and how you can offer it now. This might include sharing information, giving guidance, or leaving messages that provide comfort and clarity when they are needed most.

This kind of preparation is an act of care. It reduces uncertainty, strengthens connections, and allows you to leave behind a sense of completeness rather than unanswered questions. Approaching this part of the process with intention creates steadiness for you and for the people who will one day carry your memory forward.

Emotional preparation also creates peace. Accepting that your life is finite brings peace to you; helping your family accept that everyone's life is finite, including yours, brings peace to them.

Express final wishes

Share your values and priorities for end-of-life care so your decisions reflect who you are.

Use nonverbal communication

Even in the final stages, presence can speak more than words. Holding hands, eye contact, or quiet companionship can offer deep reassurance.

By prioritizing honesty, steady listening, and practical support, you can communicate about death in a way that is respectful, clear, and grounded.

Why silence makes things harder

Silence leads to:

- emotional unpreparedness

- isolation in grief

- poor end-of-life planning

Many people delay these conversations because they think they need all the answers first. You don't. You only need a basic understanding of your values and the direction you want to take.

These conversations are not about predicting the future. They are about creating a structure that protects your choices, reduces confusion, and gives you confidence that your wishes will be honored.

With preparation and honesty, these discussions can be straightforward, respectful, and surprisingly empowering.

By naming death, we begin to reclaim agency and intimacy with life's end.

Conversations with your primary physician

As your thoughts become clearer and you've begun sharing them with loved ones, the next step is to bring your wishes into conversations with the professionals who will help carry them out. These discussions are not emotional in the way family conversations can be, but they do require clarity and preparation. Doctors, attorneys, and financial planners each play a specific role in ensuring that your intentions are understood, documented, and legally protected.

Your primary physician will need copies of your living will and your Durable Power of Attorney for Healthcare. With these, you can also discuss:

Your current health status:

- your current conditions

- what is stable, what is worsening, and what is expected

- how your illnesses typically progress

- your prognosis, in honest, plain language

- best-case, worst-case, and most-likely scenarios

- how your health might change suddenly

- what "recovery" realistically means for your situation

Your goals and priorities

- what matters most if your health declines

- what you consider an acceptable quality of life

- what you absolutely do not want to endure

- what outcomes you value more than simply "staying alive"

Medical treatments you would accept or decline

- CPR

- mechanical ventilation

- feeding tubes

- dialysis

- surgery

- antibiotics

- blood transfusions

- treatments you would accept only if recovery is likely

When comfort should become the priority

- when you want a shift from cure-focused to comfort-focused care

- how you feel about sedation for comfort

- when hospice should be considered

- what "comfort only" means to you

Your advance directives

- your living will

- your DPOA for healthcare

- how strictly you want your written wishes followed

Your primary physician can use these documents and conversations to ensure your wishes are honored across healthcare settings.

One limitation of discussing your wishes *only* with your primary physician is that in many practices, an unfamiliar doctor may be on call during an emergency. They won't know your wishes. You and your family should keep important paperwork accessible whenever you are admitted to a hospital. Many people scan their documents and medication lists into a small, wallet-sized format.

Sustaining a practical, grounded perspective

A grounded perspective on death comes from normalizing it through conscious reflection, changing language, facing fears, and integrating mortality as a natural part of life's cycle. This helps you appreciate the present and live more meaningfully.

Key strategies include:

- engaging in end-of-life discussions

- learning from caregivers and the terminally ill

- recognizing impermanence in everyday life

- focusing on connection and legacy rather than the medical event

This transforms anxiety into motivation for a richer life.

Vignettes of people facing the end

The young mother with leukemia

"Her white blood cell count was unusually high, and further testing revealed an aggressive form of leukemia." She underwent every treatment available — chemotherapy, a bone-marrow transplant, and later an experimental T-cell therapy — but nothing halted the disease. When her physician told her that the most he could offer was time, perhaps a year, her thoughts went immediately to her infant daughter. She feared her child would grow up with no memory of her.

She began writing letters so her daughter would one day know her voice, her stories, and her love. She chose to leave the hospital and return home under hospice care, spending her final days surrounded by the people she loved most.

The sixty-two-year-old man with metastatic lung cancer

"I always thought I'd get to my real life after retirement," he said.
When he realized he wouldn't reach retirement, he didn't make a bucket list —
he made a *stop* list. He stopped pretending certain things mattered: meetings,
obligations, people who drained him. He spent his last months cooking with his
daughter, sitting on the porch, and reading the books he'd been saving. His
reckoning was a quiet reordering of priorities.

The man with ALS

"I thought reckoning with death meant some big spiritual awakening," he
told me. Instead, he found meaning in the smallest things: his wife brushing his
hair, his dog sleeping at his feet, the sound of rain on the roof. "I thought I
needed answers. Turns out I just needed to pay attention." His reckoning was
presence, not revelation.

The woman with metastatic ovarian cancer

She felt pressured to "make peace" with everyone she'd ever known. One
day she said, "I don't owe reconciliation to people who hurt me." She chose to
spend her remaining energy on the relationships that nourished her. Her
reckoning was the freedom to stop performing emotional labor she didn't owe.

The woman living fully despite terminal cancer

Told she likely had two years to live, she chose to live fully every single day.
Each morning she reminded herself, "Live a beautiful day, and then another."
Her diagnosis became a filter, sharpening her sense of what mattered and who
mattered. She didn't ignore reality — she let it clarify her life.

The woman who moved to Oregon for Death with Dignity

One woman who had been given a terminal diagnosis with less than twelve
months to live chose to live every day with purpose. Between moments hiking in
the forest, she planned a living funeral where family and friends came to dance,
laugh, tell stories, and say goodbye. She looked through boxes of photos and
reminisced. She began seeing a grief counselor. She reached out to close friends
simply to say thank you.

When she felt she was nearing the end of her life, she gave away her furniture
and clothes and moved to Oregon into a furnished rental apartment. She wanted

to use Oregon's Death with Dignity law, which allows a terminally ill patient (with a prognosis of less than six months) to request prescribed medication to bring about a peaceful death. This required two verbal requests, one written request, confirmation of prognosis and capacity from two physicians, and a fifteen-day waiting period — all while remaining in Oregon.

She said, "I'm more at peace than I've ever been."

Agnes — the eighty-two-year-old woman with incurable cancer

A doctor recently described meeting an eighty-two-year-old woman, Agnes, shortly after she learned she had an incurable cancer. Agnes had one clear wish: she wanted to stay alive long enough to finish a painting for her granddaughter's school. Her medical team arranged a gentle chemotherapy plan that eased her symptoms without causing major side effects, and for a short time the cancer quieted down. She completed the painting just as she hoped.

Not long afterward, her illness progressed again. This time, Agnes said she felt ready for the end. She chose comfort-focused care and spent the next three months with good quality of life. During her final week, she received continuous morphine, which kept her comfortable and free of significant pain. She remained awake and connected with her loved ones almost until the very end, giving and receiving heartfelt goodbyes.

Agnes approached her final chapter with clarity, purpose, and peace — a reminder that it is possible to shape the way we live, even at the end of life.

The contemporary poet

One contemporary poet has spoken openly about how receiving a diagnosis of incurable cancer reshaped her understanding of life. What might have seemed like the darkest moment instead became a profound turning point. Confronting mortality did not diminish her world; it clarified it. She described the experience as an unexpected teacher — one that revealed joy, presence, and meaning in places she had never noticed before.

Before the illness, she had lived with constant fear. Anxiety, panic, and a sense that disaster was always imminent shaped her days. Ordinary activities felt dangerous. She drank heavily, struggled emotionally, and often felt overwhelmed by the belief that life could collapse at any moment. And eventually, it did — but not in the way she had imagined.

The physical pain of cancer was immense, and at first she resisted it with everything she had. Yet at the very moment when many people feel pressured to "fight," she discovered something different: the relief of not fighting. She chose to stop resisting reality and instead allow herself to meet it where it was. That shift — simple but radical — opened a door. She described it as a moment of liberation, a sense that her entire being had room to expand.

From that point forward, time felt different. Moments became richer, fuller, more spacious. She no longer felt as though she was running out of time; instead, she felt deeply connected to the present in a way she had never experienced. The brevity of life made everything more vivid. She often said that a single moment, fully lived, could feel larger than years spent in fear.

Looking back, she realized how much of her life had been spent resisting the truth of her own circumstances. Letting go of that resistance felt like receiving a gift. It softened her view of others as well. She saw how many people on spiritual or self-improvement paths were striving desperately to "arrive" somewhere new. But the lesson she had learned was the opposite: peace comes not from striving, but from releasing. Not from adding more, but from loosening the grip on fear.

In the final stretch of her life, she expressed a simple, powerful truth: she loved her life. Accepting her illness and mortality had not taken anything away from her. It had illuminated everything. When you truly understand how brief life is, the ordinary becomes extraordinary.

Dr. Bryant Lin

Dr. Bryant Lin, a respected primary care physician and program director at Stanford Medicine, received a devastating diagnosis: Stage IV lung cancer that had already spread to his liver, bones, and brain. He had never smoked. At age fifty, he was told that the targeted drug he started might help for only a couple of years.

Instead of stepping back from his work, Dr. Lin chose to turn his illness into a teaching tool. He created a ten-week course in which he walked students through his cancer journey in real time — showing scans, describing treatments, and speaking openly about fear, pain, and uncertainty. The class filled instantly, with students crowding into the room or following online when they couldn't get a seat.

Dr. Lin explained that he wanted future physicians to understand what patients live through. Years earlier, he had received a letter from a dying patient who thanked him for treating him "like family." That message shaped his belief that medicine is, at its core, a human relationship. His course became a final lesson in that spirit.

As his illness progressed, Dr. Lin documented the physical and emotional toll — weight loss, bone pain, chemotherapy side effects, and the disorienting shift from doctor to patient. Even so, he continued to care for his own patients and mentor students. He hoped that some of them would go on to improve cancer care, and that all of them would carry forward a deeper sense of empathy.

In his teaching, Dr. Lin emphasized honesty, humility, and presence — qualities he believed mattered as much as any medical intervention. His final gift to his students was not clinical knowledge, but a lived example of how to face mortality with clarity, generosity, and purpose.

Part IV — PREPARING YOUR LEGAL AND PERSONAL DOCUMENTS - AND YOUR AFFAIRS

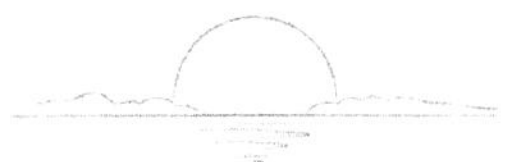

If you do not have a Will or plan for your estate, then the government has a plan for you. — Shez Christopher

Death is not the end. There remains the litigation over the estate. — Ambrose Bierce

Chapter 13:

Preparing your core legal documents

Preparing your legal documents is one of the most practical and protective steps you can take for yourself and for the people you love. In this chapter, you will learn how to talk with your doctor about medical preferences, how to work with an attorney if needed, and how to ensure your financial and legal plans reflect your values. The professionals you speak with—physicians, attorneys, financial planners—are there to help you translate your intentions into clear, actionable plans. These plans reduce uncertainty and give your loved ones confidence that they are honoring your wishes.

Core Legal Documents

Most people need four categories of documents:

- **Last Will and Testament**

- **Durable Power of Attorney (DPOA) for Financial Matters**

- **Advance Directives**, which include:
  - Living Will
  - Durable Power of Attorney for Healthcare (DPOA HC)

- **POLST** (Provider Orders for Life-Sustaining Treatment), if applicable

In some states, including North Carolina, the Living Will and DPOA-HC can be combined into a single document.

Taking the time to prepare these documents not only ensures that your wishes are clearly stated but also provides peace of mind for your loved ones. Proper planning prevents unnecessary legal complications, reduces financial strain, and allows family members to focus on what matters most: supporting one another and honoring your life.

You must complete these documents while you are mentally competent and able to make decisions.

Note About "Getting Everything in Order"

Almost no estate—or life—is ever completely in order. Life changes constantly. If you wait until everything is perfect, you may never take the first step. Beginning the conversation early is one of the greatest gifts you can give your loved ones. It reduces conflict, clarifies expectations, and protects relationships long after you are gone.

Many people imagine this part of the process will be complicated or overwhelming. Most of the essential steps are straightforward once you understand what they are. You do not need to complete everything at once, and you do not need to become an expert in legal or medical language. You simply need to understand the purpose of each document, what decisions it requires, and how to keep everything organized.

Last Will and Testament

A Last Will and Testament outlines how your property, possessions, and financial assets should be distributed after your death. It also names the person (or people) who will manage your estate—your **executor** or **administrator**.

You do **not** need an attorney to create a valid will if you follow your state's legal requirements for writing, signing, and witnessing it. A will can be:

- handwritten (in states that allow holographic wills)
- typed and printed

- created using a reputable online form

- drafted entirely by you

If it meets your state's rules, it is legally valid.

When You Might Want an Attorney

You may benefit from legal guidance if you:

- have a complex family situation (blended families, estranged relatives, dependents with special needs)

- own multiple properties or a business

- want to minimize tax issues

- expect family conflict

- want to create trusts or more advanced estate-planning tools

Without a written will, state laws determine how your property is divided. This often does **not** reflect your personal wishes and can lead to delays, financial burdens, and disputes among surviving family members.

What a Last Will and Testament *Does Not* Do

A will is essential, but it has limits. It does **not**:

Avoid all legal or financial steps

Your loved ones will still need to complete certain legal processes after your death.

Bypass probate

A will guides the probate court; it does not eliminate the probate process.

Cover medical decisions

A will only applies **after** death. It has no authority during serious illness or incapacity.

Prevent family conflict

A will clarifies your wishes, but it cannot guarantee agreement among family members.

Control what happens during your lifetime

A will only directs what happens after you die.

Durable Power of Attorney (DPOA) for Financial Matters

A DPOA for financial matters (DPOA-F) is a legal document that authorizes a trusted person—your **agent**—to manage your money and property **while you are alive** if you cannot do so yourself.

This is **not** the same as a healthcare DPOA.

What the Financial DPOA Allows

Your agent may:

- manage bank accounts
- make deposits and withdrawals
- write checks
- pay bills (utilities, mortgage, insurance, credit cards)
- handle investments
- manage real estate (buy, sell, rent, mortgage)
- file and sign tax returns
- apply for government benefits
- run your business
- access retirement accounts (within IRS rules)

Banks typically keep a copy of the DPOA-F on file once they accept it. They then treat the agent as a stand-in for the account owner. The account owner remains the sole owner; the agent simply has authority to act.

After death, the agent's authority ends immediately. The bank freezes the account until a joint owner, Payable-on-Death (POD)/Transfer on Death (TOD) beneficiary, or executor is identified.

Special Powers That Must Be Explicitly Written

Some powers are **not** automatically granted. They must be specifically included:

- making gifts
- changing beneficiary designations
- amending or creating trusts

What a Financial DPOA Cannot Do

Your agent cannot:

- make healthcare decisions

- change your will or rewrite your estate plan

- act after your death (unless named separately as executor or trustee)

When Authority Begins

You choose whether the DPOA becomes effective:

- **immediately upon signing**, or

- **only if you become incapacitated**, which requires a doctor's certification

Why a Financial DPOA Matters

A well-crafted DPOA ensures:

- your bills get paid

- your assets are protected

- your family avoids court delays

- you maintain control over who manages your affairs

You do not need an attorney to create a DPOA if you follow your state's requirements for signatures, witnesses, and notarization. However, legal guidance is recommended if you have complex finances or want to avoid mistakes that could limit your agent's authority.

A strong DPOA can also prevent the need for guardianship later—a far more expensive and stressful process for families.

The financial DPOA expires at the principal's death, at which point legal authority shifts to the executor of the Last Will and Testament or court-appointed administrator.

Advance Directives: Living Wills, Healthcare Proxies, and Medical Decision-Making

Advance Directives are the documents that guide your medical care when you cannot speak for yourself. They include:

- **Living Will**

- **Durable Power of Attorney for Healthcare (DPOA-HC)**

- **POLST**, if applicable

These documents work together to ensure that your values—not the fears, assumptions, or disagreements of others—shape your care.

You do not need an attorney to complete basic Advance Directives, though legal guidance can be helpful for complex situations. Most states provide their own forms and have specific rules for signing and witnessing. AARP and other reputable organizations offer free, state-specific documents.

Even young adults should complete these forms. Younger people often have more at stake: if they experience a catastrophic illness or accident, medical technology may keep them alive for decades in a state they would never have chosen. Every adult needs an Advance Directive.

What an Advance Directive *Does Not* Mean

Many people misunderstand what these documents do. Clarifying these misconceptions prevents confusion later.

- **Naming a healthcare proxy does not mean giving up your right to make your own decisions.**
  If you can speak for yourself, your voice is the only one that matters.

- **An Advance Directive does not mean "Do not treat."**
  It means "Treat me according to my values."

- **You must give your Advance Directive to your doctor every time you are admitted.**
  Hospitals do not automatically have access to your previous records.

- **Advance Directives are not only for older adults.**
  They are for anyone who wants their wishes respected.

Living Will

A Living Will states your preferences for medical treatment in specific, serious situations—typically when you are terminally ill, permanently unconscious, or unable to interact meaningfully with others.

The more specific your Living Will is, the more useful it becomes. Vague statements like "no heroic measures" leave too much room for interpretation.

Clear, concrete instructions—"If X happens, do Y"—give your loved ones and your medical team the guidance they need.

A Living Will is like a seatbelt. It cannot prevent every injury, but it can minimize harm.

Your Voice Still Comes First

If you can speak for yourself, your wishes override anything written in your Living Will. People often imagine how they would feel in a hypothetical situation, but when they are living it, their perspective may change. Your real-time voice always takes precedence.

Why Some Living Wills Fail

Living Wills often fall short because:

- people do not think through their wishes in detail

- they do not anticipate how complicated medical situations can become

- they never discuss their wishes with loved ones

- the document is too vague to guide real-time decisions

A Living Will is not an iron-clad guarantee of what will happen. It is a tool—one that supports your loved ones when they speak with your medical team. It is most effective when paired with a well-chosen healthcare proxy and clear conversations.

State-Specific Variations

Not all states treat Living Wills the same way.

- **Michigan and Massachusetts** do not formally recognize Living Wills as distinct legal documents. They rely instead on a healthcare proxy.

- **Religiously affiliated hospitals** may decline to follow certain instructions if they conflict with institutional policies, though they must arrange a transfer if they cannot honor your wishes.

- As of May 2025, **Alabama, Indiana, Kansas, Michigan, Missouri, South Carolina, Texas, Utah, and Wisconsin** have specific requirements for execution, witnessing, and validity.

Because of these variations, it is best to use your state's official forms or a reputable state-specific template.

End-of-Life Interventions to Consider in a Living Will

A Living Will can specify which treatments you would accept, decline, or allow only under certain conditions. These decisions fall into several categories.

1. Life-Sustaining Treatments

These are high-stakes interventions that keep the body alive when it cannot sustain itself.

A. Cardiopulmonary Resuscitation (CPR)

CPR is a medical procedure used to restart the heart and breathing.

Options include:

- Accept CPR

- Decline CPR

- Accept only if recovery to meaningful awareness is likely

B. Breathing Tube / Mechanical Ventilation

Intubation involves placing a tube through the mouth, past the vocal cords, and into the trachea. Because the tube passes through the vocal cords, the patient cannot speak. Wrist restraints are often used to prevent accidental removal. Mechanical ventilation then assists or replaces breathing.

Options include:

- Accept short-term ventilation

- Decline long-term ventilation

- Decline ventilation entirely

- Accept only if recovery to independent breathing is expected

C. Artificial Nutrition and Hydration

Artificial nutrition provides calories, protein, fluids, vitamins, and minerals when a person cannot eat. It can sustain life for months or years.

Methods include:

- **Enteral feeding** (through the stomach) via a tube through the nose or a surgically placed tube through the abdominal wall
- **Parenteral nutrition** (through a vein)
    - requires a central line
    - carries risks: infection, sepsis, collapsed lung, blood clots

Options include:

- Accept short-term feeding tube
- Decline feeding tube
- Decline artificial hydration
- Accept only if recovery is expected. What would meaningful recovery look like for you?

D. Dialysis

Dialysis filters the blood when the kidneys fail. ICU dialysis requires a large-bore central venous catheter that carries significant risks.

Options include:

- Accept dialysis
- Decline dialysis
- Accept only if temporary and reversible

E. Intravenous Fluids

IV fluids provide hydration but not nutrition. Without nutrition, a person may survive 1–3 weeks depending on health and illness severity.

2. Medical Treatments for Serious Illness

These are common in hospitals and ICU care.

A. Surgery

- Accept if it improves comfort (to decrease pain or symptom management)
- Decline if it only prolongs dying
- Accept only if it restores meaningful function

B. Antibiotics

- Accept for acute infection

- Decline if they only prolong dying

- Accept all antibiotics without restriction

C. Blood Transfusions

- Accept

- Decline

- Accept only if part of a reversible condition

D. Surgical Tracheostomy

A tracheostomy creates a surgical airway in the neck. It is often considered when intubation exceeds 10–14 days to prevent airway damage.

Options include:

- Accept if it improves comfort

- Decline if it only prolongs dying

- Accept only if it restores meaningful function

3. Comfort-Focused Care

These treatments prioritize relief of suffering.

A. Pain Management

Accept all medications necessary for comfort, even if they may unintentionally shorten life.

B. Medications for Anxiety, Agitation, or Breathlessness

Accept medications for comfort, including sedation if needed.

C. Hospice and Palliative Care

- Request hospice when eligible

- Request palliative care at any stage of serious illness

4. Situations Where These Wishes Apply

You can specify that your choices apply when you are:

- permanently unconscious

- unable to interact meaningfully with others

- in the end stages of a terminal illness

- dependent on machines with no reasonable chance of recovery

- living with advanced dementia and unable to recognize loved ones

5. Your Personal Definition of an Acceptable Quality of Life

This is where your values guide your care.

Examples include:

- "I do not want life-prolonging treatment if I cannot be mentally aware and able to interact."

- "I decline treatments that extend biological life without restoring meaningful function."

- "I want comfort to be the priority if full recovery is unlikely."

Not everyone fears physical decline in the same way. Some people value mental clarity above all else. Others prioritize physical independence. Values are deeply personal, and assumptions—especially by clinicians—can be wrong.

One patient once said, "My mind is my life to me; I don't care about my body." He wanted full resuscitation despite severe illness. His clarity rearranged the room. It reminded everyone that values are not universal.

Communicating your priorities turns your values into actionable guidance. It gives your family and care team a compass.

What a Living Will Does — and Does Not — Do

A Living Will is legally binding in theory, but in real clinical environments, several forces collide. Understanding these forces helps you appreciate why documentation alone is not enough—and why conversations with loved ones and your healthcare proxy matter just as much.

Physicians Fear Legal Liability

Many clinicians, rightly or wrongly, fear being sued. Lawsuits for withholding treatment are extremely rare, but the cultural belief persists that physicians are safer if they "do everything." This fear is cultural, not legal, yet it shapes behavior.

Hospitals Are Risk-Averse

If even one family member is distressed and demanding treatment, hospitals often continue aggressive care until the conflict is resolved. This:

- buys time

- avoids confrontation

- protects the institution

A Single Family Member Can Create Chaos

Even if your wishes are documented, one relative saying:

"You can't let him just die."

…can trigger:

- ethics consults

- administrative delays

- physicians defaulting to aggressive care

- postponement of withdrawal of life support

Vague Living Wills Create Loopholes

Statements like "no heroic measures" or "no machines" are too open to interpretation. A distressed family member can exploit that ambiguity.

Emotional Pressure Is Enormous

In moments of crisis, a document in a chart feels abstract compared to the raw emotion of a family member pleading for more time.

Why a Living Will Is Not a DNR

You could have ten Living Wills on file, but if your heart stops and there is **no physician's order** in the chart stating:

"Do Not Resuscitate (DNR)"

…the medical team is legally and ethically required to perform full resuscitation.

A Living Will **supports** your loved ones when they say:

"My father didn't want this."

If the attending physician agrees that the document reflects your wishes, they must then write an official DNR order. Without that order, full resuscitation is mandatory.

The Limits of Predicting the Future

There are countless shades between full health and severe illness. Living Wills cannot anticipate every scenario. They often lack the specificity needed for real-time decisions, which is why they rely on:

- your family
- your healthcare proxy
- your documented values

…to interpret what you would truly want.

If you appoint a DPOA-HC, it is wise to inform your family ahead of time and address disagreements before that authority is ever needed.

State-to-State Variations and Portability Issues

Living Wills are not universally recognized in the same way across states. Variations include:

- execution requirements
- witnessing rules

- terminology

- treatment-specific clauses (e.g., artificial nutrition)

Even if a state *technically* honors out-of-state documents, some hospitals and nursing homes may refuse to follow them due to risk aversion.

Legal Requirements Often Include:

- **Testamentary capacity:** You must understand the decisions you are making.

- **No undue influence:** You cannot be coerced or threatened.

- **Execution formalities:** Most states require signatures and witnesses; some require notarization.

- **Pregnancy clauses:** Some states suspend a Living Will during pregnancy, even if the fetus cannot survive.

From the Author

A personal note: I want to share something from my own planning that may help you think through yours. My husband is my primary Durable Power of Attorney for Healthcare, but he isn't in the medical field and doesn't really understand the complexities of medicine or ICU care. I worry that if I were unable to speak for myself—even in the event of a massive stroke from which I would not fully recover (and 'fully' is the operative word)—he might agree to any invasive intervention simply because he wouldn't know any better.

For that reason, I've named a second Durable Power of Attorney for Healthcare in my living will (it is legal in every state to add a secondary DPOA). Because she is listed in my documents, she will have access to my chart and be able to speak directly with my physicians and nurses. She is medically knowledgeable and understands the realities of nursing and medicine. She cannot override my husband's decisions, but she can help him understand what is happening and guide him toward the choices I have clearly said and documented that I want.

I sat down with them both and explained, in very specific terms (in paragraphs below), that if I cannot speak for myself, I want nothing done. If I can speak for myself, I will choose the treatments I want at that time.

My living will is lengthy, and I include it here not because you must agree with my choices, but because I have seen too many patients suffer simply because their families did not know what they wanted. If you want every possible intervention, then that is what you should choose. But choose it clearly, specifically, and in writing, so your DPOA or family members truly understand what you want—and what you do not want.

My Living Will and DPOA-HC

(I combined these two documents; many estate planning experts recommend combining a Living Will with a DPOA for healthcare matters to ensure your healthcare wishes are honored in the broadest range of circumstances).

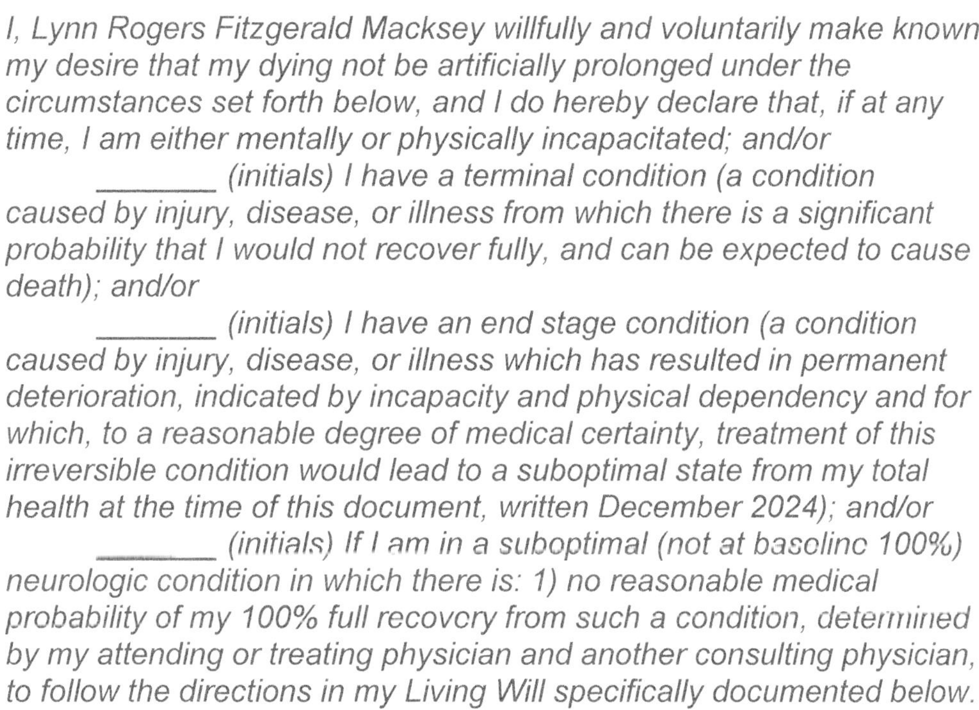

I, Lynn Rogers Fitzgerald Macksey willfully and voluntarily make known my desire that my dying not be artificially prolonged under the circumstances set forth below, and I do hereby declare that, if at any time, I am either mentally or physically incapacitated; and/or

________ (initials) I have a terminal condition (a condition caused by injury, disease, or illness from which there is a significant probability that I would not recover fully, and can be expected to cause death); and/or

________ (initials) I have an end stage condition (a condition caused by injury, disease, or illness which has resulted in permanent deterioration, indicated by incapacity and physical dependency and for which, to a reasonable degree of medical certainty, treatment of this irreversible condition would lead to a suboptimal state from my total health at the time of this document, written December 2024); and/or

________ (initials) If I am in a suboptimal (not at baseline 100%) neurologic condition in which there is: 1) no reasonable medical probability of my 100% full recovery from such a condition, determined by my attending or treating physician and another consulting physician, to follow the directions in my Living Will specifically documented below.

Designation of Surrogates
In the event that I am determined to be unable to provide informed consent regarding the withholding, withdrawal, or continuation of life-prolonging procedures, I designate the following person as my primary surrogate to carry out the provisions of this declaration:
***Name:** Keith XXXXXXXXX*
***Relationship:** Husband*
***Address:** XXXXXXXXX*
***Cell Phone:** XXXXXXXXX*

END-OF-LIFE WISHES AND BODY DISPOSITION of Lynn Rogers Fitzgerald Macksey
To my family, my physicians, my nurses, my attorney, any medical facility involved in my care, and anyone who may be called upon to make decisions regarding my health and welfare:

I was a neuro/open-heart/cardiac intensive care registered nurse for twenty-three years before attending the University of Pittsburgh to earn my master's degree in nursing with a specialty in anesthesia. Those many years in the ICU showed me the countless ways a person can come close to death or die. I have also seen this in the operating room. Death itself never troubled me as much as the patients who were resuscitated into a suboptimal state and kept alive by machines. Many were elderly, frail, and burdened with multiple comorbidities.

I once was required to give CPR on a very elderly woman from a nursing home who looked like a baby sparrow without feathers. I broke every rib in her body. What was the goal? To "save" her so she could continue living in a suboptimal state in a nursing home? It made me sick.

I have watched families grieve deeply yet be unable to let their loved one go, even when the body was clearly ready to die. I have cared for patients who lay intubated, with tubes draining every bodily function, wrists tied to prevent them from pulling at the lines, clearly in pain. Every ICU nurse I know has said, "There are worse things than death." I have cared for thousands of patients, and many times I stood at the bedside and prayed, "Please don't let this happen to me." It has always been my greatest fear to die intubated and tied to a bed.

If I am confused and say I want to live, that confusion should not override what I have written here. However, if I can clearly tell you my address, my social security number, and the phone number of where we lived in 1965 (XXXXXXXXX), and I tell you I want to live, then please treat me.

As I write this, I am sixty-nine years old. I still work, drive, paint, play piano, visit friends, and travel. But after forty-four years of caring for critically ill patients, I hurt every day from arthritis throughout my body. Some days I feel like I am 110 years old. I also live with the ordinary challenges of life. I have a history of depression and anxiety, both well-managed with medication, and I function quite well. But even with good health, the full mobility of all four limbs, and independence, I struggle. I do not want to suffer or live without these basic abilities.

Everyone defines a meaningful life differently. For me, living in a suboptimal state—anything less than what I am or can do <u>now</u>—is not acceptable. I believe in quality of life, not the quantity.

To be clear: I am not trying to die, and I am not suicidal. I married my soulmate and raised two wonderful children. I have dear friends. The people I love know this completely. I have tried to live with authenticity and kindness, and I hope, in some small way, I've made the world a better place. I have lived a full and meaningful life, achieving more than I ever imagined; I am at peace with dying when it is my time.

Therefore, if I cannot speak for myself, and if there is no hope of fully recovering to a mentally and spiritually aware, physically active, and sentient life, I DO NOT WANT ANY LIFE-SUPPORTING OR LIFE-SUSTAINING MEASURES, including:

- *CPR*
- *Intubation or mechanical ventilation*
- *Crystalloid or colloid IV fluids*
- *Blood or blood products*
- *Tracheostomy*
- *Arterial lines, central venous lines, or dialysis catheters*
- *Nasogastric or feeding tubes (enteral nutrition)*
- *Total parenteral nutrition (TPN)*
- *Surgery or invasive procedures*
- *Antibiotics*
- *Renal dialysis*
- *Any other means or devices intended to artificially maintain bodily functions*

If I can speak for myself, I will tell you what treatment I will accept
.

I often joke that you get "one good shot" at the Heimlich maneuver—if it doesn't work, let me drop to the floor. But I am not joking when I say I want to be allowed to die if I become a para-quadriplegic, if I suffer significant burns, or if I am so severely injured that I would spend months in an ICU. No thank you. Let me die in peace. I do not want to be a financial or emotional burden on the people I love, and I do not want to endure painful treatments. If you are caring for me and you would not want to endure what I am enduring, please honor my wishes.

I helped both of my parents die. I explained to their physician my philosophy for medicating a dying patient—what I call the Furrow Factor. If a patient's brow is furrowed, even with a respiratory rate of 4 (normal respiratory rate is 12-20 breaths/minute but narcotics slow the respiratory rate), it indicates they are uncomfortable and should receive medication. When my father was dying, he was conscious but breathing laboriously, frowning, and fighting the oxygen mask. I requested morphine. The physician ordered it without limitation. He needed only two small doses over about an hour, and he died without restlessness. I believe he died comfortably and in peace. That is what I want. I am not asking anyone to break the law.

I do ask for a Medlocked peripheral IV (no continuous IV fluids) so pain and anxiety medications can be given intravenously as needed to ease my suffering, even if doing so may hasten my death. If I ask for ice cream—even if my blood glucose is 900—give me ice cream (I do not want nutrition or a feeding tube). If my mouth is dry, please wet my lips and tongue or give me a sip of water for comfort. I would prefer to die at home, but if that is not possible, I want family and friends to be allowed to visit without restriction.

I beseech you to honor this directive.

After I Have Died
♥ Please give any belongings my children or husband do not want to women in need.
♥ I wish to be cremated; I do not want to be buried in a casket.
♥ I would like my ashes scattered where I scattered my mother's—at the butterfly garden XXXXXXXXXXXXXXXXXXXXXX. If possible, scatter them while it is snowing.
♥ If anyone chooses to hold a memorial service, please tell stories and laugh about all the foolish things I did and said throughout my life.
♥ And please know that I always tried my very best. I have always hoped to leave the world a better place.

Substitute decision-makers' legal priority if the patient cannot speak for themselves and no other proxies named.

- Court-appointed guardian and with healthcare decision-making authority

- Durable Power of Attorney for healthcare matters (DPOA-HC)

- Spouse

- A majority of your reasonable available parents and adult children (greater than 18 yrs old)

- A majority of your reasonable available adult brothers and sisters (greater than 18 yrs old)

- Your attending physician can make decisions after consulting with another physician if no family is available

Vignettes: When Living Wills Help — and When They're Missing

Stories often illuminate what legal documents alone cannot. These vignettes reflect patterns seen repeatedly in clinical practice: clarity brings peace, while uncertainty creates conflict, delays, and suffering.

Vignette: When a Living Will Exists to Guide Care

Patient: David, 79

Setting: ICU

David collapsed at work. Coworkers called 911, and paramedics found him without a pulse. They began CPR, delivered shocks, and placed a breathing tube. His heartbeat returned during transport, and he was admitted directly to the ICU. His wife and daughter arrived quickly and brought his Living Will. They told the ICU team that David had always been clear: he did not want to be kept alive on machines.

When they entered his room, David was somewhat awake and able to nod. They explained what had happened and asked whether he wanted the breathing tube removed, even though doing so might mean he would die. David nodded again.

The respiratory therapist removed the tube while his family held his hands. About fifteen minutes later, David took his last breath. His wife and daughter later said they were grateful that his wishes were honored and that he did not suffer long.

Vignettes: When No Living Will Exists

These stories show what happens when wishes are unclear or undocumented.

Vignette: Unclear Wishes

Patient: Mrs. A., 82
Setting: Medical floor → ICU

Mrs. A. was admitted with severe pneumonia. She lived independently but had multiple chronic illnesses. She had never completed a Living Will, and her two adult children had never discussed her wishes with her.

When her breathing worsened, the team recommended ICU transfer and possible intubation. Her children disagreed—one wanted "everything done," the other believed she would not want machines. With no documentation and no designated decision-maker, the physician defaulted to full intervention.

Mrs. A. was intubated and transferred to the ICU. She survived the initial crisis but never regained the strength to breathe on her own. After three weeks, the family agreed to withdraw life support, but the conflict left lasting emotional strain.

Vignette: Rapid Decline

Patient: Mr. J., 70
Setting: Emergency Department → ICU

Mr. J. arrived after a large stroke. He could not speak or make decisions. His wife believed he had completed a Living Will years earlier, but no document could be found, and he had never designated a healthcare proxy.

As his condition worsened, the team recommended aggressive ICU care. His wife hesitated, unsure what he would want. Extended family urged her to "fight," adding pressure and guilt. With no written guidance, the team proceeded with full treatment.

Despite maximal intervention, Mr. J. never regained consciousness. His wife later said the hardest part was not the decision to withdraw life support—it was the uncertainty of never knowing whether she honored his wishes.

Vignette: Family Disagreement

Patient: Ms. T., 65
Setting: Medical floor → ICU

Ms. T. was admitted with a severe COPD exacerbation. She had told friends she did not want to be kept alive on machines, but she had never documented her wishes.

Her three adult children arrived with conflicting views. One insisted she would never want a ventilator. Another believed she would want every possible treatment. The third felt unable to decide.

With no legal document and no appointed surrogate, the physician followed the most conservative path: full resuscitation and ICU transfer.

Ms. T. was intubated and placed on a ventilator. She remained dependent on it and developed complications. After multiple family meetings, the children finally agreed to transition to comfort care. They later expressed regret that they had not discussed her wishes earlier.

Durable Power of Attorney for Healthcare (DPOA-HC)
(also called healthcare proxy, healthcare surrogate, healthcare agent)

A DPOA-HC is a legally binding document that designates a trusted person to make medical decisions when you cannot speak for yourself. This person is authorized to:

- interpret your Living Will

- apply your values to situations not explicitly addressed

- speak with physicians and nurses

- ask questions

- clarify treatment options

- advocate for your wishes

This document covers **all** healthcare decisions—not just end-of-life care.

Key Principles

- Family members do **not** share equal authority unless they are formally named as co-agents.

- Disagreements among relatives do **not** override the agent's legal authority.

- The agent's role is to represent **your** wishes, not their own preferences.

Choosing an Agent Is Only the First Step

The real work happens in the conversations that follow. Your agent needs to understand what:

- matters most to you

- you fear

- you value

- you consider an acceptable quality of life

- you would never want

These conversations give your agent the clarity and confidence to act compassionately and decisively.

If You Choose Someone Outside Your Family

Make sure your loved ones know whom you've chosen and why. Transparency prevents confusion and reduces conflict. If tensions arise, bring your family and your agent together so they can hear directly from you.

Share Your Documents

Provide your primary physicians with:

- your Living Will

- your DPOA-HC

- the names and contact information of your agents

Bring these documents to every hospital admission. Your agent should carry them as well.

Without a DPOA-HC, decisions may fall to the court. This process is slow, stressful, and expensive—and the court-appointed guardian may not understand your wishes.

Provider Orders for Life-Sustaining Treatment (POLST)

A POLST is a medical order—not a legal document or considered an advance directive—designed for people who are seriously ill or frail. It translates your goals into **specific, actionable medical orders** that emergency personnel and healthcare providers must follow.

Key Features

- **Portable:** Travels with you across care settings.

- **Actionable:** Functions like a prescription.

- **Signed by a clinician:** Physician, NP, or PA.

- **For the seriously ill:** Not intended for healthy individuals.

- **Covers critical decisions:**
  - CPR
  - ventilation
  - feeding tubes
  - hospital transport
  - other life-sustaining treatments

A POLST is created through a shared decision-making conversation between you (or your surrogate) and your clinician. It complements—but does not replace—your Advance Directives.

Closing the Chapter

This chapter has covered the essential documents that protect your wishes and guide your care:

- Last Will and Testament

- DPOA for Financial Matters (DPOA-F)

- Living Will

- DPOA-HC

- POLST

Together, these documents form a framework that reduces uncertainty, prevents conflict, and ensures that your values—not fear, confusion, or institutional default—shape your care.

Chapter 14:

Important personal documents and your affairs

By this point in your planning, you have clarified your values, begun meaningful conversations, and identified the principles that will guide your decisions. You have already addressed the core legal documents, but there is still essential work to do: organizing personal papers, preparing your digital life, planning your funeral or memorial, and making decisions about burial or cremation.

Preparing your personal affairs is an act of consideration. It prevents unnecessary stress, reduces the burden on loved ones, and ensures that your intentions are understood—even in the smallest details. When your life is organized, your absence becomes easier for others to navigate.

This chapter focuses on gathering essential documents, organizing digital accounts, identifying important financial and household information, and making thoughtful decisions about your belongings—whether they are valuable, sentimental, or simply part of daily life. It also guides you in leaving behind the information others will need so your wishes are clear, legally recognized, and easy to follow. The goal is simple: to leave order rather than confusion.

When someone dies, it is often the everyday details—not the formal paperwork—that create the most uncertainty. Passwords no one can find. Accounts no one knew existed. Sentimental items with no instructions. Messages that were meant to be shared but never written down. Preparing your personal affairs reduces that confusion and allows the people you care about to navigate your absence with confidence instead of guesswork.

If your funeral preferences, cremation or burial choices, and other end-of-life decisions have not been discussed, your loved ones will be left to make these choices on your behalf. By talking about them now, you ensure those decisions reflect your wishes and spare your family unnecessary stress or conflict during an already difficult time.

Practical planning is not about anticipating every scenario. It is about creating a clear, reliable framework that reduces confusion and supports the people who will one day act on your behalf. When your affairs are in order, you gain peace of mind, and those you care about gain clarity.

None of this requires dramatic decisions—only attention, intention, and a willingness to put things in order while you can do so calmly.

Organizing Your Personal Documents and Digital Assets

The first step is to create a simple, intuitive structure for your information. A good system has two qualities:

- It is easy for you to maintain.

- It is easy for others to understand.

Create Master Categories

Most people find it helpful to group their information into a few broad categories:

- Personal and legal documents

- Financial and investment records

- Digital assets

- Household and practical information

- Shopping and subscription accounts

Share Access With More Than One Trusted Person

Do not rely on a single individual to locate or manage your documents. Life is unpredictable. Choose **several** trusted family members or friends who can access your papers or close accounts if needed.

Clear communication ensures your wishes are understood and reduces uncertainty for your family.

Checklist of Essential Information

Below is a comprehensive checklist to help you gather and organize what your loved ones will need. You do not need to complete everything at once. Work through it steadily and update it as your life changes.

1. Personal & Legal Documents

- ☐ Birth certificate
- ☐ Social Security card
- ☐ Passport
- ☐ Marriage certificate / divorce decree
- ☐ Property deeds
- ☐ Vehicle titles
- ☐ Life insurance policies
- ☐ Home/auto insurance policies
- ☐ Will (accessible, not stored in a safe-deposit box)
- ☐ Trust documents
- ☐ Durable Power of Attorney (financial)
- ☐ Health Care Proxy / Advance Directive
- ☐ Funeral or cremation pre-planning documents
- ☐ Organ donation information

2. Financial & Investment Records

- ☐ Bank account list
- ☐ Retirement accounts (401k, IRA, RRSP, etc.)
- ☐ Brokerage accounts
- ☐ Pension information
- ☐ Loan documents
- ☐ Mortgage or lease
- ☐ Tax returns (last 3–7 years)
- ☐ Financial advisor contact
- ☐ Accountant contact

3. Digital Assets

- ☐ Email accounts
- ☐ Cloud storage accounts
- ☐ Social media accounts
- ☐ Online banking logins
- ☐ Subscription services
- ☐ Digital photo libraries
- ☐ Domain names or websites
- ☐ Password manager location (not the password itself)
- ☐ 2-factor authentication backup codes (stored securely)

4. Household & Practical Information

☐ Utility accounts (electric, gas, water)
☐ Internet and cable accounts
☐ Cell phone provider
☐ Home maintenance contacts (plumber, electrician, HVAC)
☐ Vehicle maintenance records
☐ Pet care instructions
☐ Medication list
☐ Medical providers list
☐ Pharmacy accounts
☐ Memberships (AAA, AARP, gym, clubs)

5. Shopping & Subscription Accounts

☐ Amazon
☐ Costco / Sam's Club
☐ Pharmacy shopping accounts
☐ Streaming services (Netflix, Hulu, etc.)
☐ Auto-renewing subscriptions
☐ Loyalty programs
☐ Payment method list (no card numbers)

Creating a Storage System

Your system should be **accessible, organized**, and **secure**. Most people use a combination of physical and digital storage.

Physical Binder (Accessible in an Emergency)

Include:

☐ Last Will and Testament
☐ DPOA for financial matters
☐ DPOA for healthcare matters
☐ Living Will
☐ Insurance policies
☐ Pre-planned funeral/cremation documents
☐ A one-page "Where Everything Is" summary

Digital Folder

Stored on a flash drive kept inside the binder or in a secure home safe.

Include:

- ☐ Scans of all important documents
- ☐ Account lists
- ☐ Copies of receipts or warranties
- ☐ Inventory of digital assets

Password Manager

Store:

- ☐ Logins
- ☐ Passwords
- ☐ 2-factor authentication backup codes

(Never write passwords in the binder.)

Other Storage Tools

- ☐ Safe-deposit box inventory
- ☐ Home safe inventory
- ☐ "Where Everything Is" master index completed
- ☐ Executor or trustee informed of all locations

A Note on Commercial "Information Storage Systems"

You may see TV or TikTok ads selling personal-information binders or pre-labeled folders. These can be helpful for people who feel overwhelmed by organizing from scratch, but they are not necessary. A simple binder, a flash drive, and a password manager accomplish the same goal—often more effectively and at a lower cost.

Chapter 15:

Celebrating a life: Before death

Living Funerals

In the United States, living funerals have grown steadily in popularity over the last twenty years. As attitudes toward death shift and baby boomers seek more control over their end-of-life experiences, this practice has become increasingly familiar. Yet the idea itself is far from new. In many cultures, gathering with loved ones to say goodbye, repair relationships, and celebrate a life while the person is still present is a tradition that stretches back centuries.

In this country, a living funeral—sometimes called a prefuneral, farewell celebration, or living wake—is a gathering held for someone who is still alive, often when they have been diagnosed with a terminal illness or are nearing the end of life due to age. It is a chance for the individual to celebrate their life with the people who matter most, while they are still able to hear stories, share memories, and express final thoughts.

Too often, during a memorial service or funeral, people say they wish the honoree had been there to experience it. Many have said, "I want to hear all the nice things people might say about me at my actual funeral." A living funeral makes that possible. It allows loved ones to gather, share food, laugh, dance, tell stories, and offer the kind of heartfelt reflections that are usually spoken only after someone is gone.

Key Aspects of a Living Funeral

A living funeral is deeply personal and can be shaped in any way that feels meaningful. Common elements include:

- **A personalized celebration**
  The individual being honored often plays a central role in planning the event, choosing the tone, the setting, and the people they want present.

- **Connection and presence**
  Loved ones can speak directly to the person, offering gratitude, forgiveness, stories, and affection. The honoree can share their own reflections, hopes, and messages.

- **Emotional closure**
  These gatherings allow for meaningful goodbyes, easing the emotional burden for both the individual and their family and friends.

- **Shared memories**
  Attendees may tell stories, show photos, create a "This Is Your Life" presentation, or simply sit together and talk.

There are no rules. A living funeral can be formal or casual, structured or spontaneous, quiet or joyful. It can take place in a home, a backyard, a community center, a place of worship, or anywhere that feels right.

At its heart, a living funeral is a powerful way to celebrate a life lived, while also creating space for connection, gratitude, and closure.

For those seeking ideas or guidance, there are online resources—including step-by-step suggestions—on how to plan a living funeral.

Other Ways to Celebrate a Life Before Death

A living funeral is only one way to honor a life while the person is still present. Many people find comfort, meaning, or closure through smaller, more intimate rituals. These can be planned by the individual, by loved ones, or collaboratively.

There is no single "right" way to do this. What matters is that the experience reflects the person's values, personality, and relationships.

Below are several forms of pre-death celebration that families often find meaningful.

Legacy Projects

Some people feel called to create something that will outlive them. These projects can be simple or elaborate, private or shared.

Common legacy projects include:

- Writing letters to children, grandchildren, or friends

- Recording audio or video messages

- Creating a memory book with photos and stories

- Documenting family history

- Writing down recipes, traditions, or personal philosophies

- Organizing artwork, journals, or creative work

- Creating a "values statement" - a short reflection on what mattered most in life

Legacy projects give loved ones something to hold onto - something that carries the person's voice, humor, wisdom, and presence long after they are gone.

Gatherings of Gratitude

Not everyone wants a full living funeral. Some prefer smaller gatherings focused on gratitude, connection, or closure.

These might include a:

- dinner with close friends

- family storytelling night

- quiet afternoon with music and shared memories

- circle where each person expresses something they appreciate about the honoree

- spiritual or religious ritual

- simple backyard gathering with no agenda at all

These moments often become some of the most cherished memories for everyone involved.

One-on-One Conversations

For some people, the most meaningful goodbyes happen privately.

These conversations may include:

- forgiveness

- gratitude

- reassurance

- shared memories

- final messages

- expressions of love that were never spoken aloud

Many people say these conversations brought them more peace than any formal ceremony.

Creative Rituals

Some individuals choose symbolic acts that reflect their personality or beliefs:

- planting a tree

- creating a piece of art together

- writing messages on stones or paper

- assembling a playlist of meaningful songs

- cooking a favorite meal as a family

- taking a final trip to a beloved place

These rituals can be joyful, reflective, or both.

Celebrations of Everyday Life

Not every pre-death celebration needs to be solemn or ceremonial. Sometimes the most meaningful moments are the simplest:

- watching a favorite movie

- sharing a bottle of wine

- sitting on the porch together

- listening to music

- looking through old photographs

- laughing about the stories that always get told

These ordinary moments often become extraordinary in hindsight.

Why These Celebrations Matter

Celebrating a life before death offers something traditional funerals cannot: **presence.**

The person is there to:

- hear the stories

- feel the love

- receive gratitude

- offer their own reflections

- say what they need to say

- witness the impact of their life

For loved ones, these gatherings reduce regret. They replace "I wish I had told them…" with "I'm so glad I did."

For the person nearing death, they offer a sense of completion — a chance to see the full arc of their life reflected through the eyes of the people who knew them best.

Planning a Living Funeral or Pre-Death Celebration

A living funeral does not need to be elaborate. It does not require a script, a theme, or a perfect plan. What it needs—more than anything—is intention. The purpose is connection, not performance.

Still, a little structure can help the gathering feel comfortable and meaningful for everyone involved.

Below are gentle guidelines to help shape the experience.

1. Start With the Person's Values

The most important question is simple:

What would feel right to the person being honored?

Some people want a joyful celebration with music, food, and laughter.
Others prefer a quiet, intimate gathering with only a few loved ones.
Some want to speak; others want to listen.
Some want a spiritual or religious element; others do not.

Let the person's personality guide the tone:

- Are they sentimental or humorous?

- Do they love big gatherings or small circles?

- Do they enjoy storytelling, music, or ritual?

- Do they prefer structure or spontaneity?

A living funeral should feel like *them*.

2. Decide Who Should Be There

This is not a traditional funeral where everyone who ever knew the person might attend. A living funeral is more personal.

The honoree may choose:

- immediate family

- close friends

- a few colleagues

- spiritual or community leaders

- no one outside the inner circle

Some people want to invite everyone who has shaped their life. Others want only the people who know their heart.

There is no wrong choice.

3. Choose a Setting That Feels Comfortable

Living funerals can take place anywhere:

- home or backyard

- favorite restaurant

- community center

- place of worship

- park or garden

- beach or lake

- hospice gathering room

The setting should feel safe, familiar, and accessible for the honoree.

4. Create a Gentle Flow (Optional)

Some gatherings unfold naturally. Others benefit from a loose structure, such as a:

- welcome or opening reflection

- slideshow or "This Is Your Life" moment

- storytelling or open sharing

- reading or music played

- blessing, prayer, or moment of silence

- toast

- closing message from the honoree

This is not a performance. It is simply a way to help people feel oriented and comfortable.

5. Include Elements That Bring Joy

Small touches can make the gathering feel deeply personal:

- favorite foods or desserts

- a playlist of meaningful songs

- photos from different stages of life

- a memory table

- a guest book or message jar

- a video recording (if the honoree wants it)

- a shared ritual, like lighting candles or planting a tree

These elements help transform the gathering into a celebration rather than a farewell.

6. Prepare for Emotions — All of Them

Living funerals are beautiful, but they can also be emotionally intense. People may:

- laugh

- cry

- freeze

- feel awkward

- feel grateful

- feel overwhelmed

- feel relieved

All of this is normal.

It can help to gently remind attendees:

- there is no "right" way to feel.

- tears are welcome.

- laughter is welcome.

- silence is welcome.

The goal is authenticity, not composure.

7. Support the Honoree

The person being celebrated may feel:

- deeply moved

- tired

- energized

- vulnerable

- joyful

- overwhelmed

It helps to:

- keep the event a manageable length

- provide a quiet space for breaks

- assign someone to check in with them

- avoid surprises unless they specifically want them

Their comfort is the priority.

8. Capture the Moment (If They Want)

Some people want:

- photos

- video

- audio recordings

- written messages

- a memory book

Others prefer no documentation at all. Always ask first.

9. After the Gathering

A living funeral often brings a sense of peace and completion, but it can also stir emotions for days afterward. Loved ones may want to:

- share additional stories
- write letters
- spend quiet time together
- revisit old memories
- offer practical support

The gathering is not an ending — it is a beginning of a new phase of connection.

When Someone Is Uncomfortable With the Idea

Not everyone wants a living funeral. Some people feel:

- *shy*
- *overwhelmed*
- *private*
- *afraid of being the center of attention*
- *uncertain how to respond emotionally*

If the honoree is hesitant, consider alternatives:

- *a small dinner*
- *a quiet afternoon with a few loved ones*
- *one-on-one visits*
- *a legacy project*
- *a letter-writing circle*
- *a shared ritual without a large gathering*

The goal is not to force a celebration but to create space for connection in whatever form feels right.

Cultural and Spiritual Variations

Many cultures have long traditions of honoring a person before death:

- Buddhist and Hindu communities may hold blessing ceremonies.

- some Indigenous cultures gather for storytelling and communal support.

- Irish wakes historically included both mourning and celebration.

- Japanese *kanreki* and *beiju* celebrations honor elders at milestone ages.

- African and Caribbean traditions often blend music, prayer, and communal storytelling.

A living funeral can draw from these traditions or stand entirely on its own.

The Heart of It All

A living funeral is not about death.
It is about **presence**, **connection**, and **gratitude**.

It is a chance to say:

- "Thank you."

- "I love you."

- "You mattered."

- "Your life touched mine."

And for the honoree to say:

- "I see you."

- "I hear you."

- "I am grateful."

- "I am at peace."

These moments become some of the most cherished memories families carry forward.

Letters, Messages, and Ethical Wills

Not every expression of love or closure needs to happen in a gathering.
Many people find comfort in leaving behind written or recorded messages—gifts that can be opened later, when loved ones need them most.

These messages do not need to be long or poetic. They simply need to be sincere.

Legacy Letters

Legacy letters are personal messages written to specific people—children, grandchildren, partners, and friends. They often include:

- memories
- gratitude
- hopes for the future
- blessings or encouragement
- stories the writer wants preserved
- reflections on what mattered most

Some people write one letter for each person. Others write a single letter to be read by all. Some record audio or video messages instead of writing.

There is no wrong way to do this.

Ethical Wills

An ethical will is not a legal document. It is a statement of values—what you learned, what you believed in, what guided your life. Ethical wills often include:

- lessons learned
- personal philosophies
- spiritual reflections
- stories of resilience
- expressions of love
- hopes for future generations

These documents can be a powerful source of comfort and grounding for families long after a person has died.

Messages for Milestones

Some people choose to leave messages for future moments:

- birthdays
- graduations

- weddings

- anniversaries

- the birth of a child

- the first holiday without them

These messages can be short—a paragraph, a memory, a blessing. What matters is the presence they offer at a moment when the absence might feel sharpest.

Legacy Conversations

Not everything needs to be written down. Some of the most meaningful legacies are spoken aloud.

Legacy conversations often include what they:

- are proud of

- regret

- want their loved ones to remember

- hope for the future

- want to release

- want to forgive

- want to say "thank you" for

These conversations can be structured or spontaneous. They can happen at the bedside, on a porch, during a walk, or over a cup of tea. What matters is the honesty and presence shared in the moment.

Preparing Loved Ones Emotionally

As death approaches, families often struggle with:

- fear

- anticipatory grief

- uncertainty

- guilt

- the desire to "be strong"

- the fear of saying the wrong thing

One of the greatest gifts a dying person can offer is emotional clarity. This might include:

- reassuring loved ones that they will be okay; trust they will carry-on

- giving permission to grieve

- giving permission to live fully after the loss

- naming the people who will support them

- acknowledging the love that has shaped their life

Such conversations do not erase feelings of grief, but they soften their edges.

Talking About Death in a Natural, Loving Way

Many people fear that talking about death will make it more real. In truth, the opposite is often true. When death is acknowledged openly:

- fear decreases

- intimacy increases

- misunderstandings dissolve

- regrets shrink

- love becomes clearer

A natural, loving conversation about death might sound like:

- "I want you to know how much you've meant to me."

- "Here's what I hope for you after I'm gone."

- "I want you to keep living your life fully."

- "I'm not afraid. I'm grateful."

- "I want you to remember that you were the joy of my life."

These conversations become anchors—moments loved ones return to again and again.

When Someone Doesn't Want to Talk About Death

Some people simply cannot engage in these conversations. They may feel:

- *overwhelmed*

- *frightened*

- *avoidant*

- *protective of others*

- *emotionally unprepared*

If someone resists, it is important to honor that boundary. Instead of forcing the conversation, consider:

- *writing a letter they can read later*

- *sharing memories instead of discussing death*

- *focusing on gratitude rather than finality*

- *offering reassurance without naming the end directly*

- *Connection can happen without explicit discussion of death.*

The Gift of Presence

Celebrating a life before death is ultimately about presence—being fully with one another in a moment that will never come again.

It is about:

- saying what needs to be said

- hearing what needs to be heard

- offering comfort

- receiving love

- acknowledging the fullness of a life

- honoring the relationships that shaped it

These moments become the stories families tell for generations.

A Final Reflection: The Courage to Celebrate While You're Still Here

Celebrating a life before death requires courage — not only from the person who is dying, but from everyone who loves them. It asks us to step toward honesty rather than away from it, to choose presence over avoidance, and to embrace connection even when the future feels uncertain.

These gatherings, letters, conversations, and rituals are not about pretending death is easy. They are about acknowledging that love does not end simply because life is nearing its close. They are about creating space for gratitude, forgiveness, laughter, and truth — the things that matter most when time becomes precious.

A living funeral or pre-death celebration is not a rehearsal for loss. It is a recognition of life. It is a moment to say, this is

- *who you are to us*

- *how you shaped our lives*

- *what we will carry forward*

And for the person nearing death, it is a moment to say, I:

- *see the love around me*

- *know what my life meant*

- *am at peace*

Again, these experiences soften grief. They create memories that become anchors — reminders that even in the face of loss, there was connection, honesty, and love.

In the end, celebrating a life before death is one of the most human things we can do. It honors the truth that relationships are not defined by their ending, but by the depth of presence we bring to one another while we are still here.

Chapter 16:

Lessons to be learned from the dying

People who are nearing the end of life often see with clarity the rest of us rarely access. When the noise of daily living falls away, what remains is the essence of what mattered all along. The dying person becomes our teachers—not because they are perfect or enlightened, but because they are honest. They no longer have the luxury of pretending.

What they say, what they regret, what they cherish, and what they release can guide the rest of us toward a more intentional life.

Below are the lessons most often spoken at the bedside, in quiet conversations, in whispered confessions, and in moments of startling lucidity.

What Truly Matters

When time becomes short, priorities sharpen. People stop talking about careers, accomplishments, or the things they accumulated. Instead, they speak about the:

- people they loved

- relationships they tended or neglected

- moments that brought joy

- regrets they wish they could undo

- forgiveness they hope to give or receive

The dying remind us that life is not measured in achievements but in connection.

Dying Is the Final Developmental Stage of Life

Just as childhood, adolescence, and adulthood shape us, so does dying. It is not a failure or an interruption; it is a stage of human development. Many people use this time to reflect, reconcile, and integrate the story of their life.

Some describe it as a kind of emotional or spiritual maturation. Others see it as a return to simplicity. Either way, it is a stage with its own tasks, its own wisdom, and its own opportunities for growth.

Talking About Death Reduces Fear

People who talk openly about death—long before they are dying—tend to approach the end with more peace. Naming the truth removes its power to terrify. Avoidance, on the other hand, magnifies fear.

The dying often say they wish they had spoken about death earlier, not because it would have changed the outcome, but because it would have changed the experience.

Relationships Matter More Than Achievements

No one at the end of life talks about promotions, awards, or bank accounts. They talk about the people:

- they loved
- they hurt
- who shaped them
- they wish they had held closer

Achievements fade. Relationships endure.

Presence Is More Important Than Fixing

The dying rarely want solutions. They want presence. They want someone to sit with them, hold their hand, listen to their stories, or simply be there in silence.

They teach us that love is not measured by what we do, but by how fully we show up.

Prepare for Your Death Early — You'll Learn About Yourself

People who prepare early—emotionally, practically, and spiritually—often say the process taught them more about themselves than they expected. It clarified their values, strengthened their relationships, and helped them live with greater intention.

Preparation is not morbid. It is a form of self-knowledge.

Gratitude and Small Joys Become Central

As life narrows, the smallest joys become profound:

- sunlight through a window

- a favorite meal

- a familiar voice

- a memory retold

- a moment of laughter

- someone's hand held in silence

The dying remind us that joy is rarely found in the extraordinary. It lives in the ordinary moments we overlook.

Letting Go Can Be a Form of Strength

Letting go is not giving up. It is choosing peace over struggle. Many people reach a point where they no longer fear death—they fear prolonged suffering, unfinished conversations, or leaving loved ones unprepared.

Letting go becomes an act of love.

Life Is Finite — and That's What Gives It Shape

The dying understand something most of us forget: life's finiteness is what makes it meaningful. If we lived forever, nothing would matter. The limits of time give weight to our choices, urgency to our relationships, and beauty to our days.

The dying remind us that life is precious precisely because it ends.

Part V – WHAT YOU SHOULD KNOW ABOUT HOSPITALIZATION

In the end, the question is not just how we die—but who gets to decide?
— Unknown author

The ICU is not a temple—it is a machine. We must enter it with knowledge, not blind hope. Sometimes, the most heroic act is to stop. To choose comfort over conquest.
— Unknown author

Chapter 17:

A person's health before an acute illness or event

A person's health before a major illness or injury plays a profound role in how well they can withstand and recover from trauma or illness. This is something clinicians see every day: two patients may face the same illness, yet their outcomes can be dramatically different depending on their baseline health, their chronic conditions, and the strength of their physiological reserve.

Baseline Health and Physiological Reserve

People with fewer chronic health conditions—and those who maintain regular physical activity—tend to have healthier organs and a greater ability to recover from serious illness or injury. Their bodies have more reserve: stronger muscles, more efficient lungs, healthier blood vessels, and a heart that can tolerate stress.

In contrast, people who are less active or who live with significant comorbidities often face greater challenges. Conditions such as:

- diabetes

- heart failure

- chronic obstructive pulmonary disease (COPD)

- coronary or peripheral vascular disease

- chronic kidney or liver disease

- immune system disorders

…all reduce the body's ability to respond to sudden stress. These conditions may be stable in everyday life, but they limit how much strain the body can tolerate during a crisis.

Why People "Feel Healthy" Until They Aren't

Before a major illness, a person's organs may function well enough that they *feel* healthy—especially if nothing in daily life pushes their body beyond its usual limits. Many people never stress their heart, lungs, or muscles enough to reveal hidden problems.

But when a serious health event occurs, the entire body is suddenly placed under intense stress. Every organ system must work harder. The:

- heart pumps faster

- lungs work harder to oxygenate the blood

- kidneys filter stress hormones and medications

- liver processes toxins

- immune system activates at full force

If any organ is already weakened—even slightly—this stress can expose vulnerabilities that were invisible before.

How One Organ Affects the Others

The body is an interconnected system. When one organ begins to fail, others often follow.

For example, after a heart attack, damaged heart muscle reduces the amount of oxygen-rich blood reaching the rest of the body. Every organ depends on that oxygen. When blood flow drops, the:

- kidneys may fail

- liver may become injured

- brain may not receive enough oxygen

- lungs may fill with fluid

- blood pressure may collapse

This is how *cascading organ dysfunction* begins. It is not caused by one problem alone, but by the chain reaction that follows.

Even people with no known heart disease may have silent or mild dysfunction that causes no symptoms—until a major stress exposes it.

A Real-Life Example

I have a seventy-year-old cousin who walks six miles five days a week, stays thin, and eats a healthy diet. He believed he was very healthy—and in many ways, he was.

During a routine physical, his EKG looked abnormal. His doctor ordered a stress test, which also showed a problem. A cardiac catheterization revealed a major blockage in one of his main coronary arteries. He needed a stent to keep the artery open and maintain blood flow. Fortunately, they caught the problem before he had a heart attack, so his heart muscle remained strong. He had no idea anything was wrong.

Now imagine he hadn't known about that blockage.

Imagine he developed COVID-19, followed by pneumonia, and ended up in the ICU with a breathing tube on a ventilator. Severe illness and ICU care place enormous stress on the body. Heart rate rises. Blood pressure fluctuates. The heart must work harder than ever.

With an undiagnosed blockage, that stress could have reduced blood flow to the heart muscle, triggering a heart attack and weakening the heart enough to affect every other organ. What began as a respiratory illness could have become a multi-organ crisis.

This is the reality clinicians see every day.

Chapter 18:

A person's health after an acute illness or event

A person's health after a major illness or event depends heavily on the condition of their body before the crisis began. Patients with multiple comorbidities—such as diabetes, lung disease, heart failure, vascular disease, or chronic kidney or liver problems—often struggle long before they reach the hospital. Many already have difficulty with daily activities. When a major event like a heart attack, stroke, or severe infection occurs, ICU care may save their life, but their recovery is often limited.

Recovery Cannot Exceed the Baseline

One of the hardest truths for families to hear is this:

A person cannot recover to a better level than the health they had before the crisis.

If someone was frail, weak, or dependent before a major illness, they will not emerge stronger afterward. At best, they may return to their previous baseline. More often, they decline.

In the ICU, we frequently stabilize patients to a *suboptimal* state. They survive, but survival may require long-term support such as:

- a feeding tube

- a tracheostomy tube to maintain their airway

- dialysis

- total assistance with daily activities

A small number of patients eventually regain enough strength to enter rehabilitation, have these tubes removed, and—after many weeks or months—return home. But even then, they are often unable to do the same activities they once enjoyed.

A major health crisis depletes the body. Even returning home is less common than most families expect. Many patients remain dependent on these supports and are unable to care for themselves.

This is difficult to read, but it is an accurate description of what happens most of the time. Not all the time—there are rare "miracles"—but they are not the norm.

The Hidden Stress of Hospitalization

Procedures, surgeries, and days spent in the hospital—away from familiar routines, natural light, and restorative sleep—disrupt the body's internal balance. Even when the medical team is doing everything right, the environment itself is stressful.

Hospitalization can cause:

- shifting lab values

- fluctuating vital signs

- sleep deprivation

- disorientation

- delirium or cognitive changes

- muscle loss

- emotional distress

These effects can linger for weeks or months. In some cases, they never fully resolve.

The Bottom Line: Hospitalization Is Profoundly Stressful

Whether someone is hospitalized for an illness, an invasive procedure, or surgery with anesthesia, the experience is profoundly stressful. That stress affects the entire person—physically, mentally, and emotionally.

Even an active eighty-year-old who played tennis several times a week may face demanding rehabilitation after a major health problem. Only a small number of patients ever return to their prior level of function.

For patients who begin with moderate or poor health, the outlook is far more limited:

- many will not survive hospitalization

- those who do often recover to a much lower level of physical ability than before

This is not pessimism. It is the clinical reality that families deserve to understand.

Post-ICU Syndrome and Long-Term Effects

Surviving a major illness or ICU stay is only the beginning. Many patients experience what is known as **Post-Intensive Care Syndrome (PICS)** — a cluster of physical, cognitive, and emotional symptoms that can last for months or years. Families are often unprepared for how dramatically a person can change after hospitalization.

Physical Effects

Even a short ICU stay can cause:

- profound muscle weakness

- difficulty walking or standing

- shortness of breath

- chronic fatigue

- decreased stamina

- new dependence on mobility aids

- difficulty performing daily activities

Muscle loss in the ICU is rapid and severe. A patient can lose **10–20% of muscle mass in the first week alone,** especially if they were already frail. Regaining that strength is slow and often incomplete.

Cognitive Effects

Many patients experience cognitive changes after critical illness, including:

- memory problems

- difficulty concentrating

- slowed thinking

- confusion

- trouble with planning or decision-making

- episodes of delirium that may recur or linger

Some describe it as "feeling foggy" or "not like myself." For older adults, these changes may never be fully resolved.

Emotional and Psychological Effects

The emotional impact of critical illness is often underestimated. Patients may experience:

- anxiety

- depression

- irritability

- sleep disturbances

- nightmares

- post-traumatic stress symptoms

The ICU is loud, bright, disorienting, and frightening. Many patients remember flashes of alarms, procedures, or hallucinations. These memories can linger long after discharge.

Why "Going to Rehab" Is Not a Guarantee

Families often assume that rehabilitation will restore a patient to their previous level of function. In reality, rehab is not a cure — it is a structured attempt to regain as much strength and independence as the body will allow.

Rehab Helps, But It Has Limits

Rehabilitation can:

- improve mobility

- rebuild some muscle strength

- teach adaptive strategies

- support safe transitions home

But rehab cannot:

- reverse organ damage

- restore lost physiological reserve

- undo years of chronic illness

- return someone to a level of health they never had

Rehab works best for people who were strong and independent before their illness. For those who were already frail, the gains are often modest.

The Hard Reality

Many patients:

- never regain the ability to walk independently

- cannot return to living alone

- require long-term care

- remain dependent on feeding tubes or tracheostomy tubes

- experience permanent cognitive decline

Families are often shocked by how little progress is made, even with weeks of therapy.

Why Two Patients With the Same Illness Have Different Outcomes

Families often ask, "Why did my loved one struggle when someone else recovered?" The answer lies in the concept of **physiological reserve** — the body's ability to withstand stress.

Two patients with the same diagnosis may have completely different outcomes because of differences in:

- age

- baseline strength

- chronic conditions

- nutritional status

- mobility

- immune function

- heart and lung health

- cognitive reserve

- frailty

A strong, active person may survive a severe illness and return home.
A frail person with multiple comorbidities may not survive the same illness — or
may survive but never recover meaningful function.

This is not unfairness. It is physiology.

Preparing Families for Realistic Outcomes

One of the greatest challenges in medicine is helping families understand
what recovery truly looks like. Hope is important, but so is clarity.

Families should know:

- survival does not equal recovery

- recovery does not equal independence

- independence may never return

- long-term care may be necessary

- cognitive changes are common

- emotional changes are common

- the person may never be the same

Understanding this early helps families make decisions rooted in reality rather
than wishful thinking.

A Closing Reflection

A major illness does not simply "happen" to the body — it transforms it.
Even when the crisis passes, the effects ripple outward for months or years.
Some people regain strength and return to a meaningful life. Others do not.
Many fall somewhere in between.

The message of this chapter is not to frighten, but to prepare. When families
understand the limits of the body after a crisis, they can make decisions with
compassion, clarity, and honesty. They can support their loved one without
unrealistic expectations. And they can recognize that sometimes the kindest
choice is not to push for more treatment, but to honor the body's limits and
prioritize comfort, dignity, and peace.

Chapter 19:

The Medical Maze

Modern medicine is extraordinary. It can reverse infections that once killed millions, open blocked arteries, replace failing organs, and sustain life through crises that would have been fatal only decades ago. But this power comes with complexity. When someone enters the hospital—especially during a serious illness—they step into a system built for action, intervention, and cure. That system can save lives, but it can also sweep patients and families into a momentum they never intended.

To navigate this maze, it helps to understand how physicians think, how hospitals function, and why the default path so often leads toward "more treatment," even when the likelihood of meaningful recovery is low.

The Curative Mindset of Admitting Physicians

Admitting physicians—whether hospitalists, internists, primary attendings, or specialists—enter the picture with a specific mandate: **diagnose the problem and attempt to fix it.** Their training, identity, and professional culture are built around restoring health, reversing disease, and stabilizing acute illness. They are curative by design.

This orientation shows up in several predictable ways:

1. Their work begins with the question: "What can we do?"

Physicians are trained to look for reversible causes, order tests, start treatments, and escalate care when needed. Their instinct is to intervene—medications, procedures, consultations, monitoring—because that is how they are taught to help.

2. They initiate the medical plan

Admitting physicians set the tones for hospitalizations. They identify the primary problems, coordinate specialists, and outline steps aimed at improvement. Their focus is on action, progress, and measurable change.

3. Their professional identity is tied to saving or restoring life

Medical culture reinforces this:

- Fix the problem

- Stabilize the patient

- Extend life

- Prevent decline

This mindset is powerful and deeply ingrained.

4. They often default to "more treatment" unless told otherwise

Because their role is curative, admitting physicians may continue offering interventions as long as options exist. Even when the likelihood of meaningful recovery is low, the momentum of medicine can push toward:

- "one more procedure"

- "one more day"

- "one more attempt"

Not out of negligence, but out of habit, hope, and training.

Why the Dying Process Has Become Longer

In earlier eras, pneumonia, kidney failure, and infections often caused rapid death. Today, medical treatments can control or postpone these complications, especially in people with cancer, heart disease, or other chronic illnesses. As a result, the dying process is often extended—not because people are healthier, but because medicine can delay the final event.

This prolongation creates a new set of questions:

- Should we continue life-prolonging treatment?

- What is the goal of care now?

- What does "meaningful recovery" look like?

- What would the patient want?

These questions become central for patients, families, and clinicians.

Hospitalization in the United States: The Landscape

Understanding the medical maze also means understanding the scale of it.

One in twelve Americans experiences a hospital stay each year.

15–20% of acute hospital admissions involve an ICU stay.

ICU admission rates rise sharply with age.

Over **700,000 people** die in hospitals each year, though this number is slowly decreasing as more people choose to die at home or in hospice.

In 2000, **48%** of Americans died in hospitals; today, that percentage is lower as care options expand.

Hospitals save lives, but they also shape how many people die—often in ways that do not reflect their values.

The Intensive Care Unit (ICU): What the Numbers Mean

About **80%** of patients admitted to the ICU survive until hospital discharge. Among those survivors:

- roughly **45%** return home

- the rest go to rehabilitation centers or skilled nursing facilities

- outcomes vary widely based on age, illness severity, and comorbidities

Factors that influence ICU outcomes include:

- Illness severity and reason for admission. Patients recovering from major surgery often fare better than those with sepsis or organ failure.

- Age and comorbidities. Younger, healthier patients have better survival rates. Older adults with chronic conditions face higher mortality.

- Length of ICU stay. Stays longer than 14–21 days are associated with significantly higher mortality and long-term decline.

These numbers matter because they help families understand what ICU care can—and cannot—achieve.

The Reality of ICU Care: Powerful Tools, Powerful Consequences

Nearly everything used in the ICU—medications, machines, procedures—carries potential side effects. These interventions are often lifesaving, but they are also extremely powerful. Critically ill patients are especially vulnerable, which means even treatments intended to help can place significant strain on the body.

Medications

ICU medications can:

- raise or lower blood pressure
- affect breathing
- injure kidneys or liver
- cause confusion or agitation
- disrupt sleep
- cause profound weakness

Sedatives and pain medications can slow breathing, lower blood pressure, cause constipation, and contribute to delirium. Some patients experience cognitive changes for months afterward.

Machines and Tubes

Ventilators, central lines, feeding tubes, and dialysis machines support failing organs but also introduce risks:

- infections
- bleeding
- lung injury
- pneumonia
- blood clots
- long-term weakness
- discomfort or agitation

To tolerate the ventilator, patients often require deep sedation or even temporary paralysis, which increases the risk of severe weakness and prolonged recovery.

The Environment

The ICU environment itself is stressful:

- constant alarms

- bright lights

- frequent blood draws/painful procedures

- interrupted sleep

- wrist restraints

- disorientation

These factors contribute to delirium, exhaustion, and long-term cognitive decline.

Why ICU Care Requires Constant Reassessment

Because ICU treatments are so powerful, the medical team must continually ask: Is this intervention still helping more than it is harming?

This is the heart of ICU medicine. It is not simply about "doing everything possible." It is about balancing benefit and burden and aligning treatment with the patient's values and likely outcome.

For families, this is why goals-of-care conversations are essential. Decisions are most meaningful when they reflect what the patient would want—not just what medicine can do.

The Voices of the ICU: What Nurses See Up Close

ICU nurses witness the realities of critical illness in a way few others do. They see the daily toll of machines, medications, and procedures. They see the suffering that families rarely imagine. And they see the limits of medicine—where treatment shifts from healing to prolonging the dying process.

Their insights offer a grounded, unfiltered view of what aggressive care truly means.

"If I'm sick enough to need CPR, I'm sick enough not to want to be resuscitated to a sicker state."— *ICU Nurse*

This perspective is common among ICU clinicians. They know that CPR is not the dramatic, life-restoring event portrayed on television. They know that:

- CPR often causes broken ribs

- survival rates are low, especially for older adults

- survivors frequently emerge with worsened organ function

- many never regain independence

- the underlying disease remains unchanged

As one nurse put it, stabilizing a critically ill patient after CPR often means "resuscitating them into a sub-normal state." *How* sub-normal depends on the patient's baseline health—and sometimes, on luck.

"We can treat many things… but should we? And if yes, should we always?" — ICU Nurse

---

Modern medicine has extraordinary tools:

- chemotherapy

- dialysis

- ventilators

- vasopressors

- invasive surgeries

- experimental treatments

But every intervention has a cost—pain, side effects, complications, or prolonged suffering. ICU nurses see the cumulative burden of these treatments, especially when the underlying disease is irreversible.

They ask the questions families often don't know to ask:

- How will this help?

- How will this hurt?

- What are the risks?

- What is the likely outcome?

- What is the patient's quality of life during and after this?

These questions are not about giving up. They are about aligning treatment with reality and with the patient's values.

"What is one day worth?"— ICU Nurse

This question stops people in their tracks because it forces a reckoning.

One day can be priceless—if it is a day of connection, clarity, or comfort. But one day in the ICU, attached to machines, sedated, restrained, or suffering, may not be the day a patient would choose.

Families must decide not only **how long** someone lives, but **how** they live.

When Emotional and Spiritual Preparation Meets Medical Reality

Families often approach serious illness with expectations shaped by faith, tradition, or personal beliefs about how dying "should" unfold. They imagine:

- a peaceful transition

- time for final conversations

- the chance to say goodbye

- a quiet room, not a noisy ICU

But modern medicine does not always allow for this. Critical illness can move quickly. Machines, alarms, sedation, and rapid decisions can overwhelm even the most prepared family.

Emotional and spiritual readiness must be paired with an understanding of:

- the likely trajectory of the illness

- the limits of technology

- the implications of choosing Full Code

- what ICU care looks like

- what recovery realistically means

This alignment does not eliminate grief, but it reduces shock and regret. It allows families to make decisions that honor both the patient's values and the truth of the situation.

The Physician's Role — and the Influence of Personal Ethics

Physicians are trained to save lives. Their instinct is to act, intervene, and push forward. But modern ICU practice is slowly shifting from a reflexive "save at all costs" mindset toward a more thoughtful, patient-aligned approach.

Still, many patients receive life-prolonging interventions that offer little meaningful benefit. This often happens because:

- prognosis was not clearly explained

- conversations were rushed or avoided

- families assumed every procedure was necessary

- physicians offered interventions simply because they were possible

Every physician brings personal ethics and values into their work. Their beliefs shape how they interpret risk, choose treatments, and balance suffering, autonomy, and longevity. Two physicians may approach the same situation very differently—one leaning toward aggressive intervention, another toward comfort-focused care.

This variation is part of the humanity of medicine, but it can confuse families and overshadow the patient's own values.

This is why preparation matters.
Clear communication, advance directives, and documented wishes anchor the care plan. They reduce the influence of individual physician variation and ensure decisions reflect what the patient—not the clinician—believes is right.

Hospitals Are Built for Action, Not for Dying

Most Americans still die in hospitals. These deaths unfold within systems designed for efficiency, safety, and rapid response—not for ritual, reflection, or deeply personal decision-making.

When a patient becomes unstable, the hospital's default is action:

- call a Rapid Response

- escalate monitoring

- transfer to the ICU

- initiate life support

These steps are appropriate for reversible illness. But for patients with advanced disease or poor baseline health, these same protocols can propel them into a high-tech dying process they never would have chosen.

Unless a patient's values are explicitly documented, the system defaults to **Full Code**—even when aggressive treatment offers little chance of meaningful recovery.

Families often assume that comfort, dignity, and peace will guide care at the end of life. Unless those values are clearly communicated, they can be overshadowed by the momentum of medical routines.

The Hard Truth: Medicine Can Fight, But It Cannot Win

Atul Gawande writes:

"The waning days of our lives are given over to treatments that addle our brains and sap our bodies for a sliver's chance of benefit... We have allowed our fates to be controlled by the imperatives of medicine, technology, and strangers."

Medicine exists to fight disease. But death is not a disease. It is a certainty.

In a war you cannot win, you do not want a general who fights to the point of annihilation. You want someone who knows when to advance and when to surrender—someone who understands that fighting to the bitter end can cause more harm than good.

The essential question becomes:

What is the goal of treatment, and what is the likelihood of achieving that goal?

Chapter 20:

Hospital policies regarding resuscitation for *any* patient

When someone is admitted to the hospital, their "code status" becomes one of the most important—and least understood—parts of their medical record. Code status determines what will happen if their heart stops, if they stop breathing, or if their condition suddenly collapses. Most people assume they will have time to decide. In reality, the decision is made for them the moment they are admitted unless they have documented otherwise.

Understanding how hospitals respond to emergencies—and what each code status truly means—is essential for making informed choices about care.

How a Hospital Responds to a Sudden Decline

A patient on a hospital floor rarely goes from "fine" to "coding" in one dramatic leap. Decline can be gradual: subtle changes in breathing, blood pressure, or mental status that accumulate until the body can no longer compensate. When the tipping point comes, the bedside nurse calls for the crash cart.

No matter the underlying cause, the event is labeled a **Code**.

On the hospital floors, this triggers a specialized Code Team—physicians, nurses, respiratory therapists, pharmacists, and others—who arrive within minutes. By the time they reach the room, the bedside nurse has already begun CPR. The team works rapidly to stabilize the patient, though not every condition can be reversed. If the patient survives those first critical moments, they are rushed to the ICU for ongoing resuscitation and support.

This entire cascade happens automatically **unless the patient has a documented limitation on resuscitation**.

The Default: <u>Full Code</u>

If a patient has no advance directive, no living will, and no documented preferences, they are automatically determined to be a **Full Code**. This means:

- CPR

- defibrillation (shocks)

- intubation and mechanical ventilation

- emergency medications

- invasive procedures

- ICU transfer

Full Code is not a neutral choice. It is a commitment to every possible intervention, regardless of the likelihood of meaningful recovery.

Vignette: The Default

Mr. B., 76 — diabetes, chronic kidney disease, moderate heart failure

Mr. B. was admitted with worsening shortness of breath. He had never completed a living will, so he was automatically assumed to be a Full Code. Over the next 48 hours, his condition deteriorated. A Rapid Response was called; he was intubated and transferred to the ICU.

There, he required a ventilator, vasopressors, and dialysis. His kidneys did not recover. He remained sedated and dependent on life-sustaining treatments. When the ICU team explained his prognosis, his family was stunned—they had assumed "Full Code" meant "treat the illness," not "use every possible intervention, even if it prolongs dying."

After days of complications and no improvement, the family shifted to comfort-focused care. Mr. B. died peacefully. Later, his family expressed regret that they had never discussed his wishes with his doctor.

Vignette: Full Code at All Costs

Mrs. H., 79 — advanced dementia, chronic kidney disease, recurrent infections

Mrs. H. was admitted with sepsis. She had no living will and no healthcare proxy. By default, she was a Full Code. When her condition worsened, the team recommended against intubation, explaining that her chances of meaningful recovery were extremely low. Her children insisted on "doing everything."

She was intubated, placed on vasopressors, and treated aggressively. Over the next two weeks, she developed multi-organ failure. She died during a cardiac arrest, and because she was Full Code, the team performed CPR despite knowing it would not succeed.

After her death, her children expressed sorrow and exhaustion. One admitted they had not understood what "Full Code" truly meant.

Do Not Resuscitate (DNR / No Code)

A **DNR** order means that if the patient's heart stops or they stop breathing the healthcare team should not perform:

- CPR

- Shocks/defibrillation

- Intubation

But **full medical treatment continues** until that moment. This includes:

- antibiotics

- IV fluids

- oxygen

- medications

- surgery (if appropriate)

- hospitalization

DNR does **not** mean "do not treat." It means "do not attempt to restart the heart or breathing once they stop."

Do Not Intubate (DNI)

A **DNI** order means:

- CPR may be attempted

- shocks may be used

- medications may be given

- **but no breathing tube will be placed**

Oxygen can be given by mask, but the patient must be able to breathe on their own. CPR without the option of intubation is less likely to succeed, but honoring the patient's limits is essential.

Many people choose combinations:

- DNR but not DNI

- DNI but not DNR

- Full treatment until arrest

- Comfort-focused care only

There is no single "right" choice—only the choice that reflects the patient's values.

Why Comfort Measures Must Be Explicit

Preventing unwanted treatment is only half the equation. It is equally important to ensure that **comfort-focused care is available and ordered**. Unless the medical record explicitly includes orders for:

- pain relief

- oxygen for comfort

- anti-nausea medications

- sedation for distress

…there is a risk these essential supports may be withheld. These treatments are not "futile." They are vital for easing suffering.

Ask the attending physician to order **"comfort measures"** if comfort is the goal.

Most ICU healthcare providers know to order comfort measures, but there is nothing wrong with talking with the doctors to make sure they have done so.

Justice Sandra Day O'Connor affirmed in 1997 that patients experiencing great pain have no legal barrier to receiving pain medication "even to the point of causing unconsciousness and hastening death." Comfort is a protected right.

Hospice as a Path to Comfort (see Hospice and Palliative Care below)

Hospice care ensures comprehensive comfort-focused treatment. Even ICU patients may choose hospice if they meet criteria and decline life-sustaining machines. Hospice is not about giving up—it is about shifting the goal from cure to comfort, from prolonging life to easing suffering.

The Importance of Documentation

A DNR order must be:

* written

* signed by a licensed clinician

* placed in the medical record

At home, a state-approved DNR form must be visible—often on the refrigerator or bedside. A bracelet alone is not enough. EMS personnel **must** see the official form; otherwise, they are legally required to perform CPR, intubation, and transport.

No Code: When the Goal Is Not Resuscitation

A **No Code** (or **DNR**) order means that if the patient's heart stops or they stop breathing, the medical team will not attempt CPR, shocks, or intubation. But until that moment, the patient still receives full medical treatment— antibiotics, oxygen, fluids, medications, and any other interventions that align with their goals.

No Code is not about "giving up." It is about recognizing that resuscitation would not restore the life the patient values, and that avoiding invasive procedures is the most compassionate choice.

The following vignettes illustrate how No Code decisions play out in real hospital settings.

Vignette: No Code With Clear Goals of Care

Mrs. P., 89 — advanced heart failure and frailty

Mrs. P. had completed a living will years earlier and clearly documented No Code status. Her daughter, her healthcare proxy, understood her wishes. When Mrs. P.'s breathing worsened, the team focused on easing distress—oxygen, medications, and comfort.

When she became unresponsive, no CPR or intubation was attempted. She died peacefully several hours later. Her daughter later said the clarity of her mother's wishes made the experience calmer and less frightening.

Vignette: No Code but Full Treatment Until Arrest

Mr. K., 72 — metastatic lung cancer

Mr. K. wanted full medical treatment short of CPR or intubation. He received antibiotics, fluids, and oxygen. When he developed sudden respiratory distress, the Rapid Response team provided noninvasive support, but his condition continued to decline.

When his heart stopped, the team honored his No Code order. No CPR was initiated. His family was present and grateful that he was not subjected to procedures he had explicitly refused.

Vignette: No Code With Family Conflict

Ms. D., 81 — dementia and recurrent infections

Ms. D. had a longstanding No Code order signed by her physician and healthcare proxy. When she was admitted with sepsis, her younger daughter—who had not been involved in earlier discussions—insisted that "everything be done."

The medical team reviewed the documentation and held a family meeting. They explained that No Code meant no CPR or intubation, but that she would still receive appropriate treatment for her infection. The daughter struggled but ultimately accepted her mother's prior decision.

Ms. D. died later that evening without resuscitative efforts. Afterward, the daughter acknowledged that honoring the No Code order prevented a traumatic, invasive death.

When a Patient Chooses DNR After Aggressive Treatment

Sometimes a patient or family chooses DNR only after seeing the toll of aggressive interventions.

Vignette: From Open-Heart Surgery to DNR

Jim, 44 — lupus with severe heart valve disease

Jim underwent a second valve replacement, but the surgery went poorly. He required an intra-aortic balloon pump and multiple intravenous medications to maintain blood pressure. His kidneys began to fail. Over days, his organs deteriorated.

His wife realized that even if he survived, he would never return to the life he valued. She changed his status to DNR. Later that afternoon, with his wife and ICU nurse at his bedside, Jim's heart rate slowed. His eyes opened wide with a look of joy and wonder. Then his heart stopped.

His wife and nurse both felt he had seen something beautiful in his final moment.

Vignette: Choosing comfort when there is no choice for recovery

I was sitting with my 86-year-old father in the emergency room once he had been stabilized after a massive heart attack. He was comfortable, alert and oriented. His hospital physician came to speak with him. Both of my parents had told me multiple times over the years that if they were to become critically ill, they did not want to be put on life support. Right in front of my dad, I asked the doctor to please order that he was to be a "do not resuscitate" and "do not intubate" also known in hospital lingo as a DNR and DNI. I think he was surprised I was so direct, so he turned to my father with a raised eyebrow. his gaze quizzical but my father said, "yes, just like she said, I don't want any type of life support, invasive treatments, or surgery."

Later that afternoon, I came back to visit him and found him in extreme respiratory difficulty. I got as much information as I could from the doctor and found out his heart muscles had become too weak for him to survive. As he struggled to breathe, I was able to ask him if he wanted to change his mind about the breathing tube, as it was our only hope at this point, and he shook his head and said no. He said OK to have an oxygen breathing mask that would help push oxygen through his mouth into his lungs. He seemed to relax and he was still oriented. Several hours later, it was now 2:30 in the morning and he was struggling even more to breathe and his brow was furrowed. I wanted my dad to be as comfortable as he could possibly be. The doctor and I discussed the known effect of narcotics leading to suppressed respiration. I explained to the physician that while I was not trying to kill my father, I wanted him to be comfortable at all costs as there was no hope for his recovery. I explained that if his breathing was getting worse and his brow was furrowed, indicating that he was in pain, I wanted him to receive morphine for comfort, even if his respiratory rate was two (normal respiratory rate is 12- 20 breaths per minute). He agreed and wrote the order for morphine PRN, meaning without time restrictions or dose limit. Dad received two separate small doses of Morphine over the next hour when he struggled or grimaced, and he rested better for a while. His face relaxed much more after both doses. After the second dose he died—about 30 minutes later. No Code Blue. No emergency response/CPR/intubation/defibrillation. He died with the three of his us by his bedside, his wife, his son-in-law. and me, holding his hands.

Withdrawal of Life Support

This is not a code status. It is a planned, medically supervised decision made when treatment no longer offers benefit and only prolongs suffering. It is not about "causing death," but about allowing the underlying illness to take its natural course once artificial support is removed.

Withdrawal is appropriate when:

- recovery is no longer possible

- treatment is prolonging dying rather than prolonging living

- the patient's values prioritize comfort over invasive interventions

The focus shifts from cure to comfort, from prolongation to dignity.

Talking With a Patient Before Withdrawal

If the patient is awake or intermittently aware, simple, gentle questions can help guide care:

What matters most

- What matters most to you right now?

- Is there someone you want to see or speak with?

Comfort and suffering

- What makes you uncomfortable that we should avoid?

- What would help you feel more at ease?

Emotional needs

- Is there a message you want us to share with someone?

- Is there anything unfinished that weighs on you?

Tips for communication:

- Keep questions short.

- Use yes/no or simple choices.

- Watch for nonverbal cues.

- Ask one question at a time.

- Rephrase gently if needed.

These conversations can bring profound peace to both patient and family.

What Withdrawal of Life Support Involves

Withdrawal typically includes stopping:

- mechanical ventilation

- medications that artificially maintain blood pressure or heart rate

- dialysis

- artificial nutrition or hydration

- routine tests or monitoring

Starting comfort care with medications—opioids, sedatives, anti-anxiety medications—are used to ensure the patient does not experience distress.

Most patients die within minutes to hours after withdrawal, though some live longer depending on their underlying condition.

The process is gentle, intentional, and focused entirely on comfort.

<u>Vignettes: Withdrawal of Life Support</u>

Withdrawal After Prolonged ICU Course

Mr. L., 83 — pneumonia, chronic heart failure

After two weeks on a ventilator with no improvement, his family agreed that continued treatment would only prolong suffering. The ventilator was removed while he remained deeply sedated. He died peacefully within an hour.

Withdrawal After Devastating Neurologic Injury

Ms. J., 68 — massive intracerebral hemorrhage

Imaging showed catastrophic brain injury. Her daughters recalled her saying she would never want to live dependent on machines. Life support was withdrawn, and she died within minutes. Her daughters felt they had honored her clearly stated wishes.

Withdrawal Following Family Reconciliation

Mr. S., 59 — septic shock

His adult children initially disagreed about limiting treatment. After several meetings with the ICU team, they reached consensus. Life support was withdrawn, and he died later that afternoon. The family later said the process helped them reconcile.

From Full Code to Comfort-Focused Care

Mr. R., 74 — severe COPD, heart failure, diabetes

His sons insisted on "doing everything," not understanding what Full Code entailed. After days of complications and clear explanations from the ICU team, they shifted to comfort-focused care. The ventilator was withdrawn, and he died peacefully with both sons at his bedside.

What Code Status Really Means

Code status is not a bureaucratic detail. It is a declaration of values. It determines whether the hospital will attempt to restart a failing heart, place a breathing tube, or initiate a cascade of invasive interventions. It determines whether a person dies in an ICU surrounded by machines or in a quieter space surrounded by people they love.

Most importantly, code status determines whether the final chapter of a person's life reflects their wishes—or the hospital's defaults.

Understanding these choices before a crisis is the greatest gift a person can give their family. When wishes are clear, families are spared the agony of guessing. When documentation is in place, clinicians can act with confidence. When values are known, treatment aligns with the person rather than the system.

Choosing Wisely: Questions That Clarify Values

The right code status is not about age, diagnosis, or prognosis alone. It is about what matters most to the individual. These are clarification questions:

- What does a "good day" look like for you?

- What abilities are essential to your sense of self?

- What would you consider an unacceptable quality of life?

- How much medical intervention are you willing to undergo for a small chance of improvement?

- If your heart stopped, would you want to be resuscitated knowing the risks of brain injury, organ failure, or permanent dependence on machines?

- If recovery were unlikely, would you prefer comfort over prolongation?

These questions are not morbid. They are acts of love.

The Difference Between Prolonging Life and Prolonging Dying

Modern medicine can keep a heart beating long after the body has lost the ability to heal. It can support failing organs, replace lost functions, and sustain life through extraordinary means. But it cannot restore meaning when the underlying illness is irreversible.

The distinction is simple but profound:

- **Prolonging life** supports a body that can recover.
- **Prolonging dying** supports a body that cannot.

The challenge is recognizing which situation you are in.

Families often assume that "doing everything" is the safest choice. In reality, "everything" can mean:

- weeks of sedation
- repeated procedures
- restraints
- infections
- organ failure
- a death that is traumatic rather than peaceful

The question is not whether medicine *can* intervene, but whether intervention serves the person's values.

Why Clarity Before a Crisis Matters

When a crisis hits, decisions must be made quickly. Emotions run high. Families may disagree. Physicians may default to action. Without clear documentation, the hospital will follow its protocols—not the patient's preferences.

Clarity prevents:

- unwanted CPR
- unwanted intubation

- unwanted ICU transfers

- family conflict

- prolonged suffering

Clarity allows:

- comfort-focused care

- peaceful dying

- family presence

- dignity

- alignment with values

Advance directives, living wills, and healthcare proxies are not just paperwork—they are protection.

The Role of the Family

Families often carry the emotional weight of decisions the patient never made. They may feel guilt, fear, or pressure to "fight." They may confuse stopping treatment with giving up hope. They may not understand what resuscitation entails.

Families need to know:

- honoring a patient's wishes is not abandonment

- comfort-focused care is active, compassionate medical care

- choosing not to prolong suffering is an act of love

- the goal is not to extend life at any cost, but to honor the life that was lived

When families understand the likely outcomes, they can make decisions rooted in love rather than fear.

The Role of the Clinician

Clinicians are trained to save lives. But they are also responsible for helping patients and families understand when treatment no longer serves the patient's goals. Their role is not to decide for the patient, but to:

- explain prognosis clearly

- describe what interventions entail

- outline likely outcomes

- support values-based decisions

- ensure comfort when cure is no longer possible

The best clinicians know when to fight—and when to shift toward peace.

The Heart of the Matter

At its core, code status is not about medicine. It is about meaning.

It is about deciding what:

- kind of life is worth living.

- kind of death is acceptable?

- matters most when time becomes short?

These are not strictly medical concerns.

When people make these decisions early—before illness, crisis, fear—they shape the final chapter of their life with intention. They spare their families' anguish. They allow clinicians to provide care that aligns with their values. And they ensure that the end of their life reflects the person they have always been.

Chapter 21:

Critical care and expectations

What You Need to Know if a Loved One Is Admitted to the ICU

Few experiences are as disorienting as having a loved one admitted to the ICU. The medical complexity, the unfamiliar language, the constant alarms, and the uncertainty of each hour create a level of stress most families have never encountered. Reading this chapter now—before you ever need it, and I hope you never do—gives you a foundation of understanding that can bring steadiness during an otherwise chaotic time.

In the ICU, care is delivered by a team, not a single physician. The admitting physician coordinates the overall plan, but multiple specialists are often consulted to address different aspects of the patient's condition. Your critically ill father may have:

- a cardiologist for his heart

- a pulmonologist for his lungs

- a nephrologist for his kidneys

- a neurologist for his brain

- an infectious disease specialist for infections

- a surgeon if procedures are needed

Each specialist has partners who rotate through the ICU, so the doctor you speak with today may not be the same one you meet tomorrow. This can be confusing for families, especially when each specialist focuses on only one organ system.

This is where ICU nurses become indispensable.

ICU nurses are the constant presence at the bedside. They are there 24 hours a day, seven days a week. They hand off information from one shift to the next, track changes minute by minute, and often understand the full picture better than anyone else. Physicians rely on them to notice subtle changes, communicate updates across specialties, and advocate for the patient's needs.

Talk with the nurses. They are your anchor in a setting where everything else seems to change.

When a patient cannot direct their own care, regular meetings between the healthcare team and the family serve two essential purposes. The meetings:

- ensure everyone has the same information

- affirm the family's role in decision-making

These meetings are not a formality—they are the heart of good ICU communication.

Communication Breakdowns in the ICU

Serious illness creates a perfect storm for misunderstanding. Families arrive frightened, overwhelmed, and desperate for clarity. Clinicians speak in the language of physiology, probabilities, and protocols. Both sides want the best for the patient, yet they often interpret each other's words through entirely different lenses.

How Families Mishear Clinicians

Families tend to hear reassurance even when clinicians are trying to convey concern. Phrases like:

- "We're watching closely."

- "The next 24 hours are important."

- "He's holding his own."

…can sound hopeful, even when the medical team is signaling that the situation is precarious. Hope filters everything.

How Clinicians Misinterpret Families

Clinicians may interpret a family's hope as a request for maximal intervention, even when the family is simply trying to cope with uncertainty. When a doctor asks, "Do you want us to do everything?" families almost always say yes. What they often mean is: "Do everything that's reasonable."

But they may not know what "reasonable" means, and in their shock and sorrow, they may not ask.

Clinicians, meanwhile, hear "everything" and proceed accordingly—even when the interventions are unlikely to help.

The Problem of Medical Language

Medical jargon obscures meaning. Words like:

- stable

- critical

- responding

- not a candidate for surgery

…carry specific clinical implications but can be misinterpreted as signs of improvement or abandonment.

Families may hesitate to ask questions, fearing they will seem difficult or ungrateful. Emotions amplify the gap.

Informed Consent and Expectations

Many patients and families agree to treatments without fully understanding what those treatments involve. Consent often happens during stress, fear, or confusion. Medical terms can sound reassuring even when the situation is serious.

People may picture:

- a ventilator as temporary support, not weeks of sedation or the possibility of never having the breathing tube removed

- CPR as quick and effective, not a procedure with low success rates and high risk of injury

- "stable" as good news, not simply "not actively dying this minute"

Clinicians may assume the information was clear because it was explained. But fear and hope distort how families hear it. The result is a gap between what medicine can realistically offer and what families believe they agreed to.

True, informed consent requires:

- plain language

- repeated conversations

- time to process

- space to ask questions

When families understand what treatments mean in real life, they can make decisions that reflect their values—not assumptions.

The Right Questions During a Medical Crisis

The right questions don't require medical knowledge. They require clarity, courage, and a willingness to pause the momentum of the system long enough to ensure the care reflects the patient's wishes.

Here are the most important questions to ask when the situation is serious:

1. "What is the big picture?"

Crisis care moves fast. This question forces the team to step back and explain the overall situation—not just the latest lab result.

2. "What are we hoping for, and what are we expecting?"

Hope and expectation are not the same. This question clarifies the realistic outcome, not just the best-case scenario.

3. "Is this treatment likely to help, or is it likely to prolong suffering?"

This next question is a simple, powerful way to determine whether an intervention aligns with the patient's values.

4. "If this were your family member, what would you consider?"

Clinicians cannot decide for you, but they can share perspective. This question often opens the door to honest, compassionate guidance.

5. "What will this look like for the patient in the next hours or days?"

Families need to know what the lived experience will be—sedation, pain, procedures, or inability to communicate.

6. "What are the options if things don't improve?"

This helps families understand the next steps—including comfort-focused care—before they are forced into a rushed decision.

7. "What matters most to the patient, and how can we honor that?"

This brings the conversation back to values, not protocols. It reminds everyone that the patient—not the disease—should guide the plan.

Chapter 22:

"Do everything" and the high-tech death

In the United States, many people are not so much death-denying as deeply committed to the idea that every possible resource should be used to prolong active, healthy life — and that death should be accepted only when it is "indisputably inevitable." This belief shapes how families respond to crisis, how clinicians interpret their words, and how modern hospitals deliver care at the end of life.

In the ICU, the phrase **"Do everything"** has become a powerful emotional reflex. Families say it out of love, fear, guilt, or the belief that choosing anything less means abandoning hope. Clinicians hear it as a mandate for full intervention — ventilators, vasopressors, dialysis, CPR, and every available technology — regardless of prognosis or the patient's previously expressed values.

The result is what many call **the high-tech death**: a death shaped more by machines than by meaning.

What Families Think "Everything" Means — and What It Actually Means

Across the country, countless families face the same scenario: a loved one suffers a critical event and is rushed to the ICU. In these moments, families are overwhelmed with fear and uncertainty. When clinicians ask whether they want "everything" done, they almost always say yes.

But most families do not understand what "everything" entails.

They imagine:

- a temporary crisis

- a reversible illness

- a dramatic rescue like those portrayed on television

They rarely picture the reality:

- a sedated patient connected to multiple machines

- an inability to speak, eat, or interact

- procedures that may prolong suffering without restoring function

- a body kept alive by technology long after meaningful recovery is impossible

Without clear advance directives, "Do everything" becomes the default path — even when the likelihood of recovery is extremely low.

The Emotional Toll of "Doing Everything"

The push to "do everything" carries a heavy emotional burden. When the outcome is poor — as it often is for frail or critically ill patients — families may struggle with regret. Did we:

- prolong suffering?

- misunderstand what the doctors were saying?

- make choices our loved one would never have wanted?

These doubts can linger long after the patient has died.

Even when patients survive, the cost is high. They rarely remember the ICU procedures themselves — but they feel every moment while it's happening:

- intubation

- central lines

- chest compressions

- dialysis catheters

- repeated blood draws

- turning and suctioning the airway

- sedation and delirium

None of it is gentle. None of it is painless.

When a patient had a strong quality of life before the crisis, fighting hard for recovery makes sense. But when someone has already lived with poor health or significant decline, the equation changes. They endure the same invasive interventions, yet their chances of returning to even their previous baseline are slim.

The question becomes unavoidable:

What kind of life are we saving, and at what cost to the person who must endure the process?

Survival alone is not victory if the outcome is a life marked by greater disability, dependence, or suffering than before.

Why the High-Tech Death Happens

The high-tech death is not the result of bad intentions. It is the predictable outcome of a culture that equates:

- action with hope

- technology with salvation

- stopping treatment with giving up

Without honest conversations about prognosis, values, and the limits of medicine, "doing everything" often means doing everything *except* honoring the patient's wishes.

The ICU environment amplifies this:

- machines beeping

- tubes and monitors everywhere

- rapid-fire decisions

- multiple specialists offering fragmented information

Families are shocked by the sight of their loved one in such a vulnerable state. They are asked to make decisions they never imagined making. And without prior conversations or legal documents, the burden becomes even heavier.

Even under the best circumstances — with excellent medical care and supportive staff — the ICU is profoundly stressful. When clarity is missing, families are left uncertain about what choices truly reflect their loved one's values.

The "Heroic" Narrative and the Ethical Crossroads of Modern Medicine

Modern medicine is shaped by a powerful cultural story: the belief that the right intervention, delivered at the right moment, can pull a patient back from the brink. This "heroic" narrative celebrates rescue, technological triumph, and the idea that death is something to be fought rather than accepted.

Families often arrive in crisis assuming that more treatment is always better. Television dramas, news stories, and hospital marketing portray CPR, ventilators, and last-minute interventions as routinely lifesaving. These measures frequently prolong suffering for patients with advanced illness or poor baseline health.

Clinicians are not immune to this bias. Medical training reinforces the impulse to rescue. The fear of appearing to "do nothing" — combined with concerns about legal risk — pushes teams toward maximal intervention even when the prognosis is poor.

Decisions become technical:

- ventilators

- vasopressors

- dialysis

- CPR

The focus becomes physiology — *Can this organ be supported?* — while the ethical weight of these choices goes unspoken. The absence of a clear "no" becomes a "yes," and the system moves forward with treatments that may prolong dying rather than preserve life.

This is not a failure of compassion. It is a failure to pause and ask what matters most to the person at the center of the crisis.

Why We Say "Do Everything"

Families, clinicians, and patients all wrestle with values under pressure. Ethics is not abstract — it lives in bedside decisions made every day. The reflex to "do everything" arises from several forces, each understandable, each powerful.

1. Families Often Have Unrealistic Expectations

Popular culture has profoundly shaped how people imagine medical rescue. Television portrays CPR as a reliable lifesaver. Ventilators appear temporary. Dialysis looks routine. In reality:

- CPR rarely restores meaningful life in frail or critically ill patients

- ventilators often require deep sedation and prolonged ICU stays

- dialysis can be painful, exhausting, and may not change the outcome

In decades of ICU work, I saw hundreds of patients after CPR. Only one — a healthy 52-year-old with no prior disease — walked out of the hospital after months of recovery. Healthy people sometimes benefit from CPR. Frail, elderly, or terminally ill patients almost never do.

Families don't know this. They assume "everything" means "save them," not "prolong the dying process."

2. Physicians Feel Pressure — Emotional, Ethical, and Legal

Even clinicians who hate administering futile care must navigate the wishes of families in crisis. Imagine an emergency room filled with grief, fear, and desperation. Suggesting limits on treatment can feel like betrayal. Families may think the doctor is trying to save time, money, or effort — not trying to relieve suffering.

Physicians also fear legal consequences. Continuing aggressive treatment feels safer than stopping it, even when stopping aligns with the patient's values.

3. The System Defaults to Action

Hospitals are built for intervention. Protocols are designed to save lives. When a patient arrives unconscious, the system moves automatically:

- intubate

- start vasopressors

- place lines

- initiate dialysis

- transfer to ICU

Even when a patient has documented wishes, the system can override them if the paperwork is not immediately visible or recognized.

A Story From the Field

In *Reader's Digest*, Dr. Ken Murray described a patient in his late seventies with clear, legally valid instructions refusing life support. When he arrived unconscious after a stroke, the emergency team — unaware of his wishes — intubated him and placed him on life support.

Only after Dr. Murray arrived and reviewed the documents was life support withdrawn. The patient died shortly afterward. Despite the clarity of the paperwork, the situation triggered internal concern and even a report to authorities — later dismissed.

The lesson is stark:
Even well-prepared patients can be swept into aggressive
treatment they never wanted.

From Medical Intervention to Moral Reckoning

A troubling pattern emerges when "doing everything" becomes a reflex rather than a thoughtful choice. Suffering is prolonged. Technology overshadows wisdom. The system moves forward because no one paused to ask:

- Should we?

- Who bears the cost?

- Does this align with the patient's values?

The dazzling promise of modern medicine can obscure the truth: sometimes the kindest act is not to add more machines, but to recognize the limits of what medicine can offer.

Drawbacks of Aggressive Care

Aggressive ICU treatment can keep a patient alive in the short term, but it often comes with significant burdens — especially for those who are frail or living with multiple chronic illnesses.

These burdens include:

- **Prolonged suffering** from invasive procedures and the physical stress of critical illness

- **Low likelihood of meaningful recovery**, particularly for patients with poor baseline health

- **Loss of dignity**, as the body becomes dependent on machines

- **Loss of independence**, with many survivors never returning to their prior level of function

- **Emotional and financial strain** on families

- **Moral distress for clinicians**, who know the treatments are unlikely to help

This is the backdrop for the tension between autonomy and paternalism.

Autonomy vs. Paternalism: Who Decides, and How?

The ICU is where the tension between patient autonomy and medical paternalism becomes unmistakable.

- **Autonomy** means honoring the patient's own wishes — what treatments they want, what they refuse, and how they define an acceptable quality of life.

- **Paternalism** occurs when clinicians make decisions for the patient because they believe they know what is best.

In the pressure of critical illness, these forces collide. Families may demand aggressive treatment. Physicians may fear legal consequences. The patient's voice — often the only one that truly reflects their values — can be lost. And when a family says, "Do everything," many physicians default to paternalism — not because it's medically right, but because it feels safer.

The result can be care that prolongs suffering rather than preserves dignity.

The Gap Between What Families Understand and What Clinicians Know

Families often do not fully grasp the risks, burdens, and low likelihood of success associated with many life-sustaining treatments. Clinicians, on the other hand, can often make objective assessments based on experience:

- Will CPR restore meaningful life?

- Will a ventilator help the patient recover, or merely prolong dying?

- Is a feeding tube likely to improve quality of life, or simply extend suffering?

When the "big picture" is explained clearly, patients often choose comfort-focused care rather than aggressive treatment. But these conversations must happen early — before a crisis.

Increasingly, physicians and critical care nurses feel a responsibility to help patients understand the reality of their situation. They ask:

- What matters most to you?

- Are you hoping to reach a milestone?

- Would you prioritize comfort over longevity?

- How much intervention would you want if recovery is unlikely?

These conversations ensure that care aligns with the patient's values — not the momentum of medical technology.

Vignette: The Story of Miguel Alvarez

When 82-year-old Miguel Alvarez arrived in the ICU with severe pneumonia on top of advanced heart failure, his daughter, Sofia, insisted that "everything" be done. Machines had saved him once before. She believed they could do it again.

But this time was different. He was frailer, thinner, sleeping most of the day, forgetting names, skipping meals. His primary doctor had gently suggested palliative care months earlier, but the conversation never continued.

On his second ICU day, his oxygen levels worsened despite maximal support. The next step was intubation. Sofia assumed this was the obvious choice.

The intensivist sat with her and spoke plainly. He explained that:

- CPR in someone with her father's frailty had a very low chance of restoring meaningful life

- a ventilator might keep him alive temporarily, but was unlikely to help him recover

- a feeding tube would not reverse the underlying disease

Then he asked the questions that matter:

- What mattered most to her father?

- What had he feared?

- Would he want comfort if recovery was unlikely?

Sofia remembered her father saying, *"I don't want to be kept alive by machines. I just want to be comfortable."*

Hearing the big picture clearly — without jargon, without false promises — she realized aggressive treatment no longer aligned with who her father was.

She chose comfort-focused care.

Mr. Alvarez was moved to a quiet room, away from the alarms and machinery of the ICU. His breathing was labored but peaceful. Sofia sat beside him, holding his hand, whispering memories and gratitude. The nurse dimmed the lights and brought warm blankets. Medications eased his discomfort. His breathing slowed over the next hour, and he died gently, without the violence of CPR or the isolation of deep sedation.

Later, Sofia said she felt both grief and relief — grief for losing her father, and relief that she had honored what he had once told her in a moment of honesty: *"I don't want to be kept alive by machines . . ."*

She realized that "doing everything" had not been the right question. The right question was: What would he have wanted?

The Moral Weight of "Doing Everything"

The story of Miguel Alvarez is not unusual. It is the story of thousands of families each year who must choose between the momentum of modern medicine and the values of the person they love. The high-tech death is not a failure of love — it is a failure of clarity, timing, and cultural expectation.

When families say "do everything," they are often saying:

- "I'm not ready to lose them."

- "I don't want to feel responsible for their death."

- "I'm afraid of making the wrong choice."

- "I don't understand what the alternatives are."

These are human responses, not medical decisions. But the medical system interprets them as medical orders.

Without clear guidance, the system defaults to action — not because it is always right, but because it is what the system is built to do.

The Cost of the High-Tech Death

Aggressive treatment at the end of life can:

- prolong suffering

- increase pain

- cause delirium and fear

- lead to loss of dignity

- separate patients from loved ones

- create moral distress for clinicians

- leave families with lasting regret

And yet, the system continues to move in this direction because:

- families fear "giving up"

- clinicians fear legal consequences

- hospitals are built for intervention

- culture glorifies rescue

- conversations about dying happen too late

The result is a death shaped by machines rather than meaning.

The Turning Point: From Intervention to Intention

At some point, the question must shift from:

"Can we do more?" to **"Should we?"**

And then, more importantly:

"What would the patient want if they could speak for themselves?"

This is the moral center of end-of-life care.

When clinicians and families pause long enough to ask these questions, the path often becomes clearer. Many patients, when asked early and honestly, choose comfort over prolongation. They choose presence over procedures. They choose dignity over machinery.

But these choices require conversations that happen *before* the crisis — not in the middle of it.

The Path Forward: Clarity, Courage, and Conversation

The high-tech death is not inevitable. It is the result of silence, assumptions, and the momentum of a system built for rescue. It can be changed by:

- clear advance directives

- honest conversations about values

- realistic understanding of medical outcomes

- clinicians who speak plainly and compassionately

- families who ask the right questions

- a willingness to distinguish hope from expectation

When these elements come together, the final chapter of a person's life can reflect who they are — not what the system defaults to.

- The goal is not to deny treatment.
  The goal is to ensure that treatment **aligns with the patient's values**.

- The goal is not to hasten death.
  The goal is to **prevent unnecessary suffering**.

- The goal is not to "give up."
  The goal is to **honor the life that was lived**.

Chapter 23:

What doctors in training don't learn about death and dying

In Being Mortal, *Atul Gawande asks a question that should unsettle every clinician:* **"Why are we not trained to cope with mortality?"**

Gawande admits that his training taught him how to save lives, not how to honor the end of them. The instinct was always to escalate — more surgeries, more treatments, more time. But he came to understand that *more time is not always more life*. Sometimes, in the effort to delay death, medicine erases the person.

That realization hit me hard. I thought about the people I've loved who spent their last days in sterile rooms, disconnected from everything that mattered to them. Medicine is powerful. So is the courage to ask: **"Is this the life they would have wanted?"**

Death as an Afterthought in Medical Training

Though improving, medical education in the United States often treats death as an outlier rather than an expected part of practice. Every physician will care for dying patients, yet training around death and dying remains:

- inconsistent
- optional
- theoretical
- dependent on chance exposure

A major review of U.S. medical schools found wide variation in how death and dying are taught. Many programs offer only electives rather than required coursework. Students may graduate having never practiced an end-of-life conversation in a meaningful way.

The ancient Hippocratic tradition — "respect to prolonging life" — still shapes the culture. The default is cure, not comfort. Action, not acceptance.

The Blind Spot: Communication

Communication is one of the biggest gaps in medical training. Students report feeling *"woefully unprepared"* to:

- deliver bad news

- speak with grieving families

- explain prognosis honestly

- discuss goals of care

- sit with silence, anger, or sorrow

- avoid medical jargon

- acknowledge uncertainty

Most learn these skills on the job, in moments of crisis, with no structured guidance. The result is predictable: conversations happen too late, or not at all. Families feel abandoned or confused. Patients receive more aggressive, unwanted treatment.

The Missing Skill: Talking About Death Before a Crisis

Tufts University faculty note that doctors are generally not good at talking about end-of-life issues because they receive little structured training in how to do it well. Students encounter these conversations only by chance. If they happen to be present when a dying patient's care is discussed, they learn something. If not, they graduate without ever practicing these conversations.

This is not a small omission. It shapes the entire culture of medicine.

The Missing Reflection: Their Own Mortality

Some programs now ask students to complete their own advance directive to build empathy. But this is far from universal. Without this reflection, many new doctors:

* avoid conversations about death

* default to aggressive treatment

* feel personally threatened by a patient's decline

* experience moral distress when care becomes futile

A lack of self-awareness becomes a barrier to compassionate care.

The Missing Support: Processing Their Own Emotions

Students often see their first dead body during a clinical rotation, not in a controlled learning environment. They are rarely taught:

* how to process the emotional impact of a patient's death

* how to talk about their own reactions

* how to avoid burnout or compassion fatigue

The hidden curriculum teaches them to "be strong," which often means "don't feel."

When doctors aren't trained to deal with death, the consequences ripple outward:

* patients receive more aggressive, unwanted treatment

* families feel confused or abandoned

* conversations happen too late

* dying becomes medicalized instead of humanized

* clinicians burn out

* moral injury becomes common

How Doctors and Critical Care Nurses Approach the End of Life

Many people are surprised to learn that clinicians — especially those who work closest to life-and-death situations — often make very different choices for themselves than the general public.

Physicians and critical care nurses spend their careers witnessing the:

* limits of medical treatment

* burdens of aggressive interventions

- realities of dying in a hospital

- suffering caused by "doing everything"

This firsthand experience profoundly shapes how they think about their own final days.

Clinicians Choose Differently

Research highlighted by Dr. Ken Murray shows that clinicians are far more likely than the general public to:

- complete advance directives

- decline invasive, life-prolonging treatments

- refuse CPR when meaningful recovery is unlikely

- prioritize comfort and dignity

This stands in stark contrast to the general public, whose expectations are shaped by television portrayals where CPR and last-minute rescues succeed far more often than they do in real life.

Why Clinicians Choose Comfort

For clinicians, these realities are not theoretical. They watch:

- families struggle with impossible decisions

- patients endure invasive procedures with little chance of benefit

- the emotional and physical toll of aggressive care

- the difference between a peaceful death and a medically prolonged one

Critical care nurses have a unique vantage point. Hour after hour at the bedside, they see the:

- suffering caused by prolonged ventilation

- complications of feeding tubes and vasopressors

- distress of families who don't understand the prognosis

- stark difference between a peaceful death and a high-tech one

Many quietly acknowledge that they would not want the very interventions they provide unless there was a realistic chance of recovery.

What Clinicians Know That Most People Don't

Clinicians understand:

- the limits of technology

- the cost of unnecessary suffering

- the value of comfort and dignity

- that most people can spend their final days at home

- that hospice can provide excellent pain control and support

- that repeated hospitalizations rarely improve quality of life

When time is limited, many choose to focus on what matters most:

- visiting family

- spending time with children

- taking a long-imagined trip

- savoring meaningful moments

These choices reflect clarity — about the illness, the likely time remaining, and what aggressive treatment would realistically accomplish.

When people have that clarity, they can make decisions based on their values rather than defaulting to "doing everything."

Reclaiming the Final Part of Life

When people understand the medical system, name what matters most, and make their wishes known, they reclaim authorship of the final chapter. Instead of being swept along by hospital defaults, they shape their care according to their values.

- ## This is not about controlling death.
  It is about preserving dignity.

- It is not about giving up.

  It is about choosing how to live until the end.

- It is not about limiting care.

  It is about ensuring the care reflects the person.

- Readiness is not a moment.

  It is the result of choices made long before the crisis.

And those choices allow the end of life to reflect the same clarity and purpose that shaped life its duration.

Part VI – CARE IN THE FINAL CHAPTER OF LIFE

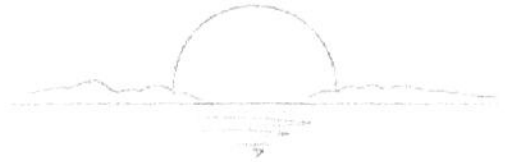

Being there for someone's last breath is a gift, but it's also something that stays with you. You don't walk away seeing life the same way again.
— Unknown author

Death is not the opposite of life, but a part of it.
— Haruki Murakami

Life and death are illusions. We are in a constant state of transformation.
— Alejandro Gonzalez Inarritu

Chapter 24:

Choosing quality of life until the end – comfort care

Almost anyone can die in peace at home. Pain can be managed better than ever. This is one of the most important truths families rarely hear early enough.

Comfort-focused care — whether delivered through palliative care or hospice — is not about giving up. It is about choosing how to live until the end. It is about shaping the final chapter with intention, dignity, and clarity. It is about replacing fear with steadiness, and medical chaos with presence.

And it begins with asking the right questions.

Asking Questions That Reveal What Matters Most

When someone is seriously ill or nearing the end of life, the most important conversations are not about lab results, ventilators, or procedures. They are about values, meaning, and what the person wants the rest of their life to look like.

These questions help families and clinicians align care with the patient's deepest priorities.

1. Questions About What Matters Most

- "What matters most to you right now?"

- "What gives your life meaning or joy?"

- "Are there people, places, or activities you want to focus on while you're here?"

These questions shift the focus from medical possibilities to personal priorities.

2. Questions About Comfort and Suffering

- "What kinds of discomfort or suffering are you most concerned about?"

- "How much pain, confusion, or difficulty breathing would be acceptable to you?"

- "Are there treatments you would rather avoid if they make you uncomfortable?"

This frames decisions around quality of life, not just longevity.

3. Questions About Medical Decisions

- "If you become very sick, what treatments would you want or not want?"
  (Examples: CPR, ventilators, feeding tubes, dialysis)

- "Would you want us to focus more on comfort or on trying every possible treatment?"

- "Are there past experiences or values that guide your choices?"

These questions help families avoid assumptions and honor the patient's voice.

4. Questions About Legacy and Relationships

- "Is there something you want to say to family or friends?"

- "Are there memories or messages you want to share?"

- "Who would you want involved in decisions if you can't speak for yourself?"

These conversations preserve connection and peace of mind.

5. Questions About Daily Comfort and Preferences

Even small choices matter:

- "Do you want visitors, and if so, who?"

- "Are there small comforts — music, books, touch — that matter to you?"

- "What makes you feel safe or calm right now?"

These details shape the emotional landscape of the final days.

- *Keep it gentle.*

- *Listen without rushing.*

- *Reflect back what you hear.*

- *Accept that answers may change.*

- *Prioritize comfort and dignity.*

These conversations are not medical tasks. They are acts of love.

What palliative care and hospice have in common

Palliative care and hospice share a common foundation: both focus on quality of life, comfort, and whole-person care. They support people with serious, chronic, or life-limiting illnesses — and they support families just as much as patients.

1. Both prioritize comfort and quality of life

They aim to relieve suffering — physical, emotional, spiritual — and help patients live as fully as possible.

2. Both support people with serious long-term illnesses

Cancer, heart failure, COPD, dementia, Parkinson's disease, and many others.

3. Both provide whole-person care

They address:

- pain

- breathlessness

- nausea

- anxiety

- depression

- spiritual distress

- family dynamics

4. Both support the family

Families receive:

- education

- emotional support

- guidance in decision-making

- help navigating the healthcare system

Illness affects the entire family unit; both models recognize this.

5. Both honor the patient's values and goals

They help patients clarify:

- what matters most

- what treatments they want or don't want

- how they want to spend their remaining time

6. Both use coordinated interdisciplinary teams

Caregivers may include:

- physicians/physician assistants (PA)

- nurses (LPN or RN)/nurse practitioners (NP)

- social workers

- chaplains

- counselors

- nurse's aides

How palliative care and hospice differ

Timing

- **Palliative care:** available at any stage of illness, from diagnosis onward.

- **Hospice:** reserved for the final months of life, typically when life expectancy is six months or less.

Goals

- **Palliative care:** can be combined with curative treatment; focuses on symptom relief and quality of life while treating disease.

- **Hospice:** focuses entirely on comfort; curative treatment has stopped.

Eligibility

- **Palliative care:** no prognosis requirement.

- **Hospice:** requires a physician to certify a life expectancy of six months or less.

Where care is provided

- **Palliative care:** hospitals, clinics, some homes.

- **Hospice:** home, hospice facilities, nursing homes, some hospitals.

Insurance

- **Palliative care:** covered like other medical specialties.

- **Hospice:** fully covered by Medicare, Medicaid, and most private insurers.

Vignette: A family choosing between palliative care and hospice

When Dr. Arjun Patel was diagnosed with advanced pancreatic cancer, his colleagues assumed he would fight it with every tool modern medicine could offer. He had spent thirty years as an oncologist urging families to "buy time" when there was still a sliver of hope.

But when he became the patient, his perspective shifted.

His tumor was metastatic. The oncologist began outlining aggressive chemotherapy and possible trials. Dr. Patel listened quietly. He knew the statistics by heart.

After the appointment, his wife asked, "What do you want to do?"

"I want to stay home," he said. "I want to feel like myself for as long as I can."

He met with the palliative care team the next day. They talked about his goals: time with grandchildren, sitting in the garden, eating real food while he still could. They adjusted medications, arranged home support, and helped him plan for what mattered most.

Over the next two months, he declined steadily but peacefully. No hospitalizations. No emergency room visits. No last-minute interventions.

He died at home, in his own bed, with his wife holding his hand.

"He wasn't being brave," she later said. "He was being honest. He knew what mattered, and he chose it."

Palliative Care: Support at Any Stage of Serious Illness

Palliative care is specialized medical care for people living with serious illnesses such as heart failure, COPD, cancer, dementia, or Parkinson's disease. Its purpose is simple: to relieve symptoms, improve quality of life, and help patients understand their treatment choices.

Palliative care can be provided:

- at any age

- at any stage of illness

- alongside curative or life-prolonging treatments

It is delivered by an interdisciplinary team — physicians, nurses, social workers, chaplains, nutritionists, and others — who work together to support the whole person.

Palliative care is not about giving up.
It is about improving life while treatment continues.

Patients often receive better:

- pain management

- emotional and spiritual support

- coordination of care

- understanding of their options

There is no eligibility requirement, no six-month prognosis, no need to stop treatment. It is a layer of support that can be added at any point in a serious illness.

Hospice Care: Comfort in the Final Months of Life

Love doesn't always mean doing everything. Sometimes it means stopping. Letting go. Sitting beside someone in the quiet and saying, "You don't have to fight anymore. I'm here."

Many families ask, "Isn't hospice giving up?"
In a healthcare system built around cure, intervention, and longevity, it's understandable that hospice is misunderstood.

But hospice is not about giving up. It is about shifting the goal of care. When cure is no longer possible — or no longer desired — hospice creates a space where:

- symptoms are managed

- comfort is prioritized

- patients can focus on what matters most

- families are supported

- dignity is preserved

Hospice staff use medical capabilities to give patients their **best possible day now**. Not to extend time at all costs, but to make the time that remains meaningful.

Hospice Can Sometimes Extend Life

Studies show that people in hospice sometimes live longer than those who continue aggressive treatment. Comfort, connection, and peace can be powerful medicine.

A hospice nurse might begin by asking:

"What is most important to you right now?"

Then she works to make that possible — adjusting medications, rearranging the room for comfort, creating routines that bring calm and predictability.

As symptoms come under control, patients often rediscover small joys: music, sunlight, a favorite food, a familiar voice. They no longer search for a way to hasten death; they look for meaning in each day.

Hospice Empowers Patients and Families

I often describe hospice as:

*the patient and family in the driver's seat, with the hospice team in the passenger's seat —
guiding, supporting, and walking alongside them.*

Time is limited, but hospice helps people use that time in ways that feel true
to who they are.

Hospice Honors the Natural Dying Process

Hospice care is:

- compassionate

- steady

- grounded in dignity

- respectful of the patient's values

It treats the whole person — physical, emotional, spiritual — and views the
family as the "unit of care."

Eligibility and Choice

Hospice is available to people with terminal illnesses and a life expectancy of
six months or less. Some people choose to continue hospitalizations and
aggressive treatments; for others, hospice offers a path that aligns more closely
with their values.

Vignettes: Care in Palliative and Hospice Settings

Vignette: The Breathless Afternoon

Mr. Alvarez, a 78-year-old man with advanced COPD, had been admitted
three times in two months for shortness of breath. Each time, the hospital
stabilized him, but he returned home weaker and more anxious.

When the palliative care team met him, he was sitting upright in a recliner,
shoulders tense, breathing fast, afraid to move.

The nurse adjusted his oxygen, gave a small dose of morphine, and coached
him through slow exhalations. Within minutes, his breathing eased. His wife,
who had been hovering anxiously, finally sat down beside him.

"This is the first time I've felt like myself in weeks," he said.

The Palliative care team didn't cure his disease.
They gave him back an afternoon — and the ability to breathe without fear.

Vignette: The Conversation at the Kitchen Table

Ms. Turner, a 64-year-old woman with metastatic breast cancer, had been avoiding conversations about her illness. Her adult children disagreed about treatment: one wanted "everything done," the other wanted comfort.

The palliative care clinician met them at the kitchen table. After listening to each person, she asked Ms. Turner what mattered most.

"I want time with my family," she said. "But I don't want to spend it in the hospital."

That single sentence shifted everything.
The family agreed to stop emergency room visits unless absolutely necessary and to prioritize comfort at home.

The conflict eased.
The patient's voice — finally spoken — became the guide.

Vignette: The Decision No One Wanted to Make

Mr. Chen, a 90-year-old man with advanced dementia, was admitted with pneumonia. He no longer recognized his daughter and had stopped eating. The medical team recommended a feeding tube. His daughter felt pressured to agree, even though she knew her father had always said he never wanted "machines keeping me alive."

The palliative care team reviewed his history, explained the natural course of dementia, and clarified that a feeding tube would not improve his comfort or prolong life in a meaningful way.

His daughter exhaled, relieved.
"I just needed someone to tell me it was okay to honor what he wanted."

She chose comfort-focused care.
Her father died peacefully a week later, without invasive procedures, surrounded by familiar voices.

Reclaiming the Final Chapter

When people hear the word *comfort*, they often imagine passivity — a kind of medical quietness, a withdrawal. But comfort-focused care is anything but passive. It is intentional, structured, and deeply human. It is a shift from fighting the illness to caring for the person. It is a recognition that the goal is no longer to add days at any cost, but to make the days that remain meaningful.

Comfort care is not about controlling death. It is about shaping life.

It is about choosing:

- presence over procedures

- connection over chaos

- dignity over machinery

- meaning over momentum

When families understand what palliative care and hospice can offer, they often feel something they haven't felt in months: relief. Relief that suffering can be eased. Relief that they don't have to navigate the medical system alone. Relief that they can focus on the person they love rather than the next crisis.

The Power of Clarity

Clarity is one of the greatest gifts in serious illness. When patients articulate what matters most — whether it's staying home, avoiding pain, seeing a grandchild, or simply being able to breathe without fear — the entire care plan shifts.

Clarity allows families to make decisions without guilt. It allows clinicians to align treatment with values. It allows the patient to remain the author of their own story.

Without clarity, the system defaults to action.
With clarity, the system can finally serve the person.

The Courage to Choose Comfort

Choosing comfort is not giving up. It is choosing how to live.

It takes courage to say:

- "I want to be home."

- "I want to be comfortable."

- "I don't want machines."

- "I want to spend my time with the people I love."

These are not medical decisions. They are human ones.

And when they are spoken aloud — when they are honored — the final chapter becomes something different from what the medical system often delivers. It becomes quieter, more intentional, more connected. It becomes a space where families can say what needs to be said, where patients can rest, where love can be expressed without the interruptions of alarms and procedures.

The Gift to Families

Families often fear that choosing comfort means abandoning hope. But the opposite is true. Comfort-focused care gives families:

- time to be present

- space to say goodbye

- confidence that suffering is eased

- reassurance that they honored their loved one's wishes

It replaces the trauma of a high-tech death with the memory of a peaceful one.

Years later, families rarely remember the exact medications or equipment.
They remember the hand they held.
The quiet room.
The final words.
The sense that their loved one was not alone.

The Heart of Comfort Care

Comfort care is not the absence of treatment.
It is the presence of the right treatment.

It is:

- pain managed well

- breath eased

- anxiety softened

- symptoms controlled

- dignity preserved

- meaning honored

It is the recognition that the end of life is not a medical failure.
It is a human experience.

And when people understand the medical system, name what matters most, and make their wishes known, they reclaim authorship of the final chapter. Instead of being swept along by hospital defaults, they shape their care according to their values.

Readiness is not a moment. It is the result of choices made long before the crisis. And those choices allow the end of life to reflect the same clarity, purpose, and love that shaped life itself.

Chapter 25:

Information for family caregivers and loved ones

Caring for someone who is dying is one of the most profound responsibilities a person can carry. It is emotional, intimate, and often overwhelming — especially when families don't know what to expect. This chapter offers a steady guide through the medical, emotional, and spiritual landscape of the final days and hours of life. Its purpose is simple: to help caregivers understand what is happening, what is normal, and how to offer comfort with confidence and love.

The Medical Aspects of Dying

As the body enters its final stage, the focus of care shifts from cure to comfort. Hospice and palliative teams work deliberately and thoughtfully to ease the physical burdens of advanced illness. Their work includes:

- managing pain and symptoms

- shortness of breath

- anxiety

- nausea

- restlessness

Medications are tailored to comfort rather than cure. The goal is not to prolong life at any cost, but to relieve suffering and support peace.

Supporting Natural Decline

The body begins to conserve energy. Families may notice:

- decreased appetite

- increased sleep

- withdrawal from daily activities

These changes are not signs of "giving up." They are part of the body's natural transition.

Coordinating Care Across Settings

Whether at home, in a facility, or in an inpatient hospice unit, the care team ensures that:

- symptoms are controlled

- the environment is calm

- the patient's comfort remains the central priority

This medical approach is grounded in the understanding that comfort — not survival at any cost — is the goal.

The Emotional Aspects of Dying

Dying is not only a physical process; it is an emotional and relational one. Hospice and palliative care teams support both the patient and the family through this transition.

Creating Space for Honest Conversations

Patients may want to express:

- fears

- regrets

- hopes

- a desire for peace

These conversations can be grounding for everyone involved.

Helping Families Understand What to Expect

Knowledge reduces fear. When families understand the signs of decline, they feel less shocked and more prepared.

Supporting Anticipatory Grief

Grief begins long before the final breath. Hospice teams normalize this, helping families understand that anticipatory grief is a human response to impending loss.

Affirming the Patient's Identity

Stories, rituals, photographs, and shared memories help anchor the patient in who they are — not just their illness.

Providing Continuity

Families are not left alone to interpret every change. Hospice teams offer reassurance, guidance, and presence.

Emotionally, hospice shifts the experience from crisis to presence. Instead of fighting the inevitable, families are guided toward understanding it, witnessing it, and finding meaning in it.

Conscious Dying and End-of-Life Rituals

Conscious dying means approaching the final stage of life with awareness, intention, and as much personal agency as possible. It does not mean controlling the moment of death. It means shaping the experience around it — physically, emotionally, and relationally — so that the patient's values guide the process.

End-of-Life Rituals

Rituals are not about prolonging life or hastening death. They provide structure and meaning during a time that can feel chaotic. They may include:

- Creating a peaceful environment: dim lights, familiar music, meaningful objects.

- Honoring relationships: shared stories, touch, presence.

- Spiritual or cultural practices: prayer, blessings, readings, symbolic gestures.

- Acts of closure: writing letters, offering forgiveness, expressing gratitude.

These rituals help families feel connected, grounded, and supported.

The Role of Caregivers and Loved Ones

Caregivers shape the final stage of life as profoundly as any medical intervention. They often become the patient's voice when the patient can no longer speak for themselves. This responsibility is meaningful — and demanding.

Practical Support

Caregivers:

- manage medications

- assist with personal care

- maintain a calm, steady environment

- coordinate with hospice teams

Emotional Support

Loved ones anchor the patient in who they are beyond their illness. Their presence — through touch, shared memories, or quiet companionship — offers connection and comfort.

Caregiving at the end of life is an act of devotion and courage. It helps shape a death that reflects the patient's dignity and values.

What Caregivers May See in the Last Days and Hours of Life

The final days of life often bring changes that can feel alarming if you don't know what to expect. These changes are not signs of failure or suffering. They are the body's natural way of shutting down — a process guided by physiology, not by choice or willpower.

Understanding these changes helps families stay steady, present, and confident.

Physical Changes

1. Decreased Appetite and Thirst

- eating becomes minimal or stops altogether

- the body no longer needs fuel in the same way

- this is normal and not a sign of suffering

Families often worry that their loved one is "starving." They are not. The body is letting go.

2. More Sleep and Less Responsiveness

- long periods of sleep

- difficulty waking

- quiet or absent responses

This is the body conserving energy. It is peaceful, not painful.

3. Changes in Breathing

- irregular breathing

- rapid breaths followed by pauses

- a soft rattling sound from the throat

The "rattle" comes from relaxed throat muscles, not distress. It is harder for families to hear than for patients to experience.

4. Cool Skin and Color Changes

- cool hands, feet, and legs

- pale or bluish skin

Circulation is slowing. This is expected.

5. Weakness and Limited Mobility

- needing help to sit up or turn

- eventually becoming bedbound

The body is conserving its remaining energy.

6. Changes in Bowel and Bladder Function

- less urine

- possible incontinence

This reflects reduced intake and kidney function.

Cognitive and Emotional Changes

1. Confusion or Disorientation

- not recognizing familiar people

- mixing up time or place

- talking about people who have died

- seeing things others cannot

- speaking of a warm light

These experiences are common and usually not frightening to the patient.

2. Withdrawal

- less interest in conversation

- turning inward

- a natural part of letting go

3. Moments of Clarity

Some people briefly become more alert:

- speaking clearly

- asking for loved ones

- sharing a final message

This can happen hours or days before death.

Communication Changes

- speech becomes softer or limited

- gestures or facial expressions may replace words

- if they cannot speak, simple cues help:
  - one blink for yes
  - two blinks for no

Even when unresponsive, **hearing is believed to remain intact**. Caregivers should continue speaking gently and reassuringly.

Emotional and Spiritual Signs

Patients may express:

- a desire to "go home"

- a sense of being "done"

- talk of traveling

- seeing loved ones who have passed

- concern for the family's wellbeing

These are normal and often comforting to the patient.

In the Final Hours

Caregivers may notice:

- longer pauses between breaths

- cool extremities

- very little urine

- eyes partially open or unfocused

- minimal or no response to voice or touch

These changes are expected. They do not necessarily indicate discomfort.

What Caregivers Can Do

- keep the environment calm and quiet

- moisten lips and gums if safe to do so

- reposition gently for comfort

- speak softly and offer reassurance

- hold their hand if touch is comforting

- allow rest without pushing food or fluids

The most important gift is presence.

The Most Important Message for Caregivers

The process of dying is not linear or orderly — and that's normal.
It moves in starts and stops. One moment the patient may be lucid; the next,
confused or silent. This unpredictability does not mean something is wrong. It is
simply how the body winds down.

Caring for someone who is dying is emotionally demanding and full of
moments that don't match the peaceful images we're taught to expect. The body
may look or behave in ways that feel alarming, but most of these changes are
natural and not painful.

*The body knows how to die.
It has its own wisdom.*

Your steady presence, calmness, and reassurance are among the greatest gifts
you can give. Even when someone cannot respond, your voice matters. Your
touch matters. Your steadiness matters.

If it seems they are holding on, they may need to know that you will be okay — that you will miss them, but you give your permission to let go. Let them know they are not alone. Offer encouragement. Tell them you love them. Share your good wishes.

These moments become the memories families carry for the rest of their lives.

Vignettes: Care for Hospice Patients

Stories help families understand what dying looks like when comfort is the goal. These vignettes illustrate the range of experiences — gradual, rapid, complex, and deeply relational.

Vignette: The Gradual Decline

Patient: Mr. L., 87 — advanced heart failure
Setting: Home hospice

Mr. L. enrolled in hospice after multiple hospitalizations left him exhausted and discouraged. Over several weeks, he slept more, ate less, and gradually withdrew from daily activities. His shortness of breath was eased with low-dose opioids; his anxiety softened with gentle reassurance and scheduled medication.

His daughter, his primary caregiver, learned to recognize the signs of decline — cool extremities, longer pauses between breaths, increasing unresponsiveness. Hospice nurses visited regularly, adjusting medications and supporting the family.

Mr. L. died quietly at home, his daughter holding his hand. Later, she said the predictability and support helped her feel prepared rather than frightened.

Vignette: A Rapid Transition

Patient: Ms. R., 72 — metastatic pancreatic cancer
Setting: Inpatient hospice unit

Ms. R. had been receiving chemotherapy until a sudden decline left her too weak to continue. She transitioned to inpatient hospice for symptom control. Her pain escalated quickly, requiring continuous medication infusions. Within days, she became less responsive.

Her family struggled with the speed of the decline, expecting more time. Hospice staff explained that rapid changes in appetite, breathing, and consciousness were part of the natural dying process.

With symptoms controlled, Ms. R. remained peaceful. She died four days after admission. Her family later said the hospice team's explanations helped them understand that the rapid decline was not a failure of care, but the final stage of her illness.

Vignette: A Complex Family Dynamic

Patient: Mr. S., 68 — end-stage COPD
Setting: Skilled nursing facility with hospice services

Mr. S. had long expressed that he did not want aggressive treatment. His adult children disagreed about limiting interventions. Hospice staff facilitated several family meetings to clarify his wishes and explain what comfort-focused care would look like.

As his breathing worsened, he became more anxious and confused. Medications eased his distress, and staff created a quiet environment to reduce stimulation. One child remained conflicted, asking whether more could be done.

The hospice nurse explained that additional interventions would prolong suffering without improving function. The family ultimately agreed to honor the patient's stated preferences. Mr. S. died with symptoms well controlled and two of his children at the bedside.

Vignette: Talking to a Dying Patient in the ICU

A patient in our ICU had been scheduled for transfer to hospice, but she began to actively die before the move. Her family hadn't arrived yet. Scott, her nurse, had cared for her for weeks. They had talked about her life, her husband who had recently died, and her fears about being alone.

Now she was unconscious, but Scott didn't want her to die without someone beside her. He sat with her, holding her hand. I heard him say softly:

"It's okay. Everything is okay. I'll talk with your family when they arrive and let them know I was with you. Go and meet your husband. When you see him, let go of my hand."

I stood outside the room and cried.

This nurse's presence was its own form of medicine.

Vignette: The Ex-Hospice Nurse Helping a Friend

Patient: Pam, 44 — metastatic cancer
Setting: Home, with hospice nurse present

Pam had been deteriorating for months. I had been a hospice nurse years earlier, and I hoped I could support Pam and her husband in an unofficial role. A month before she died, I sat on the edge of her hospital bed at home and transcribed her wishes for her funeral.

In her final week, as cancer spread to her brain, she could no longer speak but seemed to understand what was said around her. On her last evening, her husband, the hospice nurse, and I were all present. Pam became restless, trying to get out of bed.

I had been with many patients in their final hours — as an ICU nurse, as a hospice nurse — but being with a friend was different. I felt unsteady, unsure, anxious. I kept thinking, *You'd think I would be better prepared.* But I wasn't. I felt sadness, guilt, grief. I questioned whether I could have done more.

Even with experience, the heart does not follow clinical training. Love changes everything.

Author's Note — When the Patient Is Someone You Love

When my daughter was three weeks old, she developed a high fever, and we were told to take her to the emergency room. I had worked in an ER. I knew the language, the protocols, the reasons behind every test. But as the physician began listing what they needed to do, I swear I only heard every fifth word.

My fear was so overwhelming that my clinical brain simply shut down.

"Spinal tap?"
"What?"
"Blood cultures? X-rays?"

Inside, I was thinking: *This can't be happening. Not to my baby.* I was cycling through every stage of grief in minutes. My husband didn't understand anything the doctor said, and I was trying to explain it through my own panic.

What people often don't realize is that when healthcare providers have a personal relationship with the patient — especially someone who is dying — it can be just as difficult for us as for anyone else. Knowing about medicine doesn't protect us from fear or grief. Understanding the process doesn't shield us from doubt or the desperate wish for a different outcome.

Sometimes we even must guide our own family members through decisions we can barely face ourselves.

A close friend of mine, Sandi — a nurse practitioner with decades of experience — went through this with her sister, Robin. Robin had metastatic breast cancer and had clearly told her husband, Peter, that she didn't want more treatment. But when she began deteriorating rapidly, Peter didn't know he needed to ask for a Do Not Resuscitate order. He understood she couldn't be saved. He understood she didn't want more procedures. But he didn't know that without a written DNR, the default would be full resuscitation.

Sandi had to sit with him, in the middle of his heartbreak, and explain what needed to be done. Everything was happening so fast. Decisions like this often do.

Most of us in healthcare have lived through these moments with our own families. We are not immune. Knowledge does not insulate you from fear or grief when it's your own loved one.

Part VII – AFTER A LOVED ONE DIES

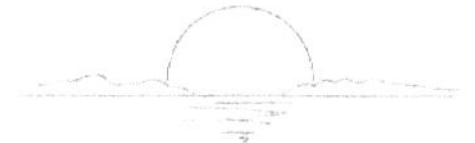

What will survive of us is love. – Philip Larkin

Death, of course, is not a failure. Death is normal. Death may be the enemy, but it is also the natural order of things. – Atul Gawande

We do not have to rely on memories to recapture the spirit of those we have loved and lost – they live within our souls in some perfect sanctuary that death cannot touch. – Nan Witcomb

Chapter 26:

Celebrating a Life: After Death

The hours and days after a death are a strange landscape — quiet and overwhelming, sacred and logistical, intimate and public. Families often feel unmoored, unsure what to do first, and surprised by how many decisions must be made quickly. This chapter offers a steady guide through the practical and ceremonial choices that follow a death, helping families shape a farewell that reflects the person's life, values, and spirit.

Some families want a traditional church funeral. Others prefer a secular celebration, a simple graveside service, or a green burial. There is no right way. There is only the way that feels true.

Church Funerals

Planning a church funeral blends logistics, tradition, and personal meaning. A clear structure helps families feel grounded during an overwhelming time and gives the service a sense of dignity and coherence.

1. Meet With the Pastor or Clergy

Most churches begin with a meeting with the pastor, priest, or minister who will lead the service. This conversation typically covers:

- the spiritual or religious tone the family wants

- Scripture readings or liturgical elements

- music guidelines (some churches limit secular songs)

- whether eulogies are allowed and how many

- any church-specific customs or restrictions

This meeting also helps clergy understand the person's life and values so the service feels authentic.

2. Choose the Type of Service

Church funerals can take several forms:

- **Traditional funeral service** (body present)
- **Memorial service** (no body present; often after cremation)
- **Mass of Christian Burial** (Catholic tradition)
- **Celebration of Life** with religious elements

3. Select Music

Music sets the emotional tone. Options may include:

- hymns meaningful to the person or family
- choir or soloist pieces
- instrumental selections
- limited secular music (depending on church policy)

Many families choose one piece for gathering, one for reflection, and one for the recessional.

4. Choose Readings

Most church funerals include:

- one or two Scripture readings
- a psalm or hymn
- optional non-scriptural readings (poems, letters, meaningful passages)

5. Plan Eulogies or Reflections

Decisions include:

- who will speak
- how long each person should talk (usually 3–5 minutes)
- whether clergy will incorporate personal stories into the homily

6. Coordinate With the Funeral Home

The funeral home and church often work together. Key decisions include:

- whether the body will be present
- open or closed casket
- timing of visitation or viewing

- transportation of the body

- flowers, guest book, printed programs

7. Decide on Ritual Elements

Depending on tradition, the service may include:

- communion

- incense

- blessings or anointing

- candle lighting

- military honors

- cultural or family rituals

8. Plan the Burial or Committal

If burial follows the service:

- coordinate timing with the cemetery

- decide who will participate (pallbearers, clergy, family)

- choose graveside readings or prayers

- decide whether the burial is public or private

Some families hold private burials and a public service.

9. Arrange a Reception or Meal

Many churches offer:

- a fellowship hall

- volunteers who prepare food

- space for photo displays or memory tables

10. Personalize the Service

Small touches can make the funeral feel like a true reflection of the person:

- photos or a memory slideshow

- favorite flowers

- meaningful objects (tools, quilts, books, medals)

- a short biography in the printed program

- a charity for memorial donations

These details help transform the service from ritual to remembrance.

Embalming

Embalming is one of the most misunderstood aspects of funeral planning. Many families assume it is required by law. It rarely is. Embalming is a temporary preservation process, not a long-term one, and it comes with environmental considerations.

Why a Body Is Embalmed

1. Temporary Preservation

Embalming slows natural decomposition for a short period — usually days, not weeks. It is helpful when:

- there will be a public viewing

- family needs time to gather

- the funeral is delayed

2. Improved Appearance for Viewing

Embalming can:

- restore color

- reduce swelling

- create a peaceful appearance

For some families, this provides comfort. For others, viewing is not important, and embalming may be unnecessary.

3. Transportation Across Long Distances

Some states or countries require embalming if:

- the body is transported across state lines

- the body is shipped by air

4. Funeral Home Policies

Some funeral homes strongly encourage or require embalming for:

- open-casket services

- extended visitations

- large public gatherings

Families can ask about refrigeration as an alternative.

5. Legal Requirements (Rare)

Embalming is legally required only in limited situations, such as:

- when burial or cremation is significantly delayed

- specific public health regulations (uncommon)

Most states allow refrigeration instead.

What Embalming Does *Not* Do

Embalming does **not**:

- preserve the body indefinitely

- prevent long-term decomposition

- sterilize the body

- improve environmental impact

Formaldehyde-based chemicals can harm soil and groundwater, which is why green burial practices avoid embalming entirely.

How Embalming Is Done (Simplified)

Arterial Embalming

A preservative solution is circulated through the vascular system while natural fluids are displaced.

Cavity Treatment

Internal organs are treated with a small amount of preservative to slow decomposition.

Restoration and Presentation

The embalmer:

- washes and dries the body

- sets facial features in a peaceful expression

- applies light cosmetics

- dresses the person

- arranges hair and positions the body in the casket

The goal is not to make the person look "made up," but to help them look like themselves.

Secular Services and Celebrations of Life

Not every farewell takes place in a church. Many people prefer a secular gathering — a celebration of life centered on meaning, memory, and personal legacy rather than religious ritual. These ceremonies can be deeply moving, highly individualized, and often feel more like a gathering of stories than a formal service.

Families choose them when the person:

- was not religious

- preferred a nontraditional approach

- wanted a celebration that reflected their personality

- valued community, creativity, or nature

Secular services offer enormous flexibility while still providing structure and emotional grounding.

1. Choose the Setting

Secular celebrations can be held almost anywhere, a:

- community center or event hall

- favorite park, garden, or beach

- private home or backyard

- restaurant, winery, or café

- workplace or club where the person spent time

The location often becomes part of the story: **"This was her favorite place to watch the sunset."**

2. Select a Facilitator

Instead of clergy, families may choose a:

- celebrant or lifecycle officiant

- close friend or family member
- funeral director trained in secular services

The facilitator sets the tone and guides the flow of the gathering.

3. Create a Structure (Flexible, Not Formal)

Secular services don't follow a fixed liturgy, but a gentle structure helps the event feel cohesive. Common elements include:

- welcome and opening reflection
- a short biography or life story
- readings (poems, letters, quotes, song lyrics)
- music meaningful to the person
- eulogies or open sharing
- a symbolic ritual (lighting candles, planting a tree, releasing flowers)
- closing words

This structure gives shape without rigidity.

4. Choose Music and Readings

Because there are no religious restrictions, families have full freedom:

- favorite songs from any genre
- excerpts from novels, letters, or journals
- quotes that reflect the person's values
- poems or lyrics that capture their spirit

These choices help the service feel personal and intimate.

5. Invite Stories and Participation

Secular gatherings often feel communal. Options include:

- open-mic storytelling
- a memory table where guests write notes
- a slideshow or video montage
- displaying artwork, quilts, tools, or hobbies
- a "toast to their life" moment

These elements help guests feel connected and involved.

6. Add a Symbolic Ritual

Symbolic acts can be powerful without being religious:

- planting a tree or scattering wildflower seeds
- releasing biodegradable lanterns or bubbles
- creating a communal art piece
- sharing a favorite food or drink
- passing around an object that mattered to the person

Rituals help mark the moment and give it emotional weight.

7. Consider a Reception or Shared Meal

Food brings people together. Families often choose a:

- potluck of the person's favorite dishes
- catered meal at a meaningful venue
- casual gathering at a brewery or café

These gatherings allow people to reconnect, share stories, and support one another.

8. Document the Event

Some families create a:

- printed program
- memory book
- digital photo album
- recording of the stories shared

These become part of the person's legacy — something future generations can hold.

Green Death and Natural Burial

A "green death" refers to an environmentally conscious approach to body care and burial. It is part of the broader green burial movement, which aims to reduce environmental impact, avoid toxic chemicals, and return the body to the earth in a natural way.

Green burial is not a single method — it is a spectrum of choices.

1. No Embalming or Nontoxic Alternatives

Green practices avoid embalming entirely or use nontoxic alternatives. This protects soil, groundwater, and surrounding ecosystems.

2. Biodegradable Materials

Bodies are placed in:

- simple wooden caskets
- woven shrouds
- bamboo, wicker, or cardboard coffins

All are designed to break down naturally.

3. Natural Burial Grounds

Green burials often occur in:

- Conservation cemeteries: burial fees support land preservation
- Natural burial forests: the body is placed directly into the earth
- Green sections of traditional cemeteries
- Recomposition (human composting): the body is transformed into soil
- Aquamation (alkaline hydrolysis): a water-based alternative to cremation

These spaces avoid concrete vaults, pesticides, and manicured lawns.

4. Minimal Carbon Footprint

Green burial reduces:

- transportation
- manufacturing of heavy caskets
- use of vaults
- energy-intensive cremation

Many families choose local burial grounds to further reduce impact.

5. Integration With Nature

Green burial sites often allow:

- native plants
- wildflowers

- trees planted as markers

- natural stones instead of headstones

The goal is to create or preserve natural habitat — a return to the earth that is simple, beautiful, and ecologically sound.

The Meaning of Green Burial

The growing interest in green burial reflects a shift in how people think about death — not as a medical event, but as a natural one. Green burial honors the body's return to the earth, avoids chemicals that harm soil and water, and supports conservation efforts.

For many families, this approach feels:

- simple

- honest

- ecological

- spiritually resonant

It is a way of saying: **"We come from the earth, and we return to it."**

Green burial is not about rejecting tradition. It is about choosing a form of rest that aligns with the person's values — environmental, spiritual, or both.

Honoring a Life in All Its Forms

Whether a family chooses a church funeral, a secular celebration, a simple graveside service, or a green burial, the purpose is the same: to honor a life with intention. Rituals — religious or not — help us mark the transition from presence to memory. They give shape to grief. They create a space where stories can be told, tears can fall, and love can be expressed without apology.

There is no single "right" way to say goodbye.
There is only the way that feels true to the person who lived. Some:

- families find comfort in hymns and Scripture. Others find it in poetry, music, or the rustle of wind through trees.

- want a crowd; others want a quiet circle of a few.

- choose a traditional burial; others choose to return the body to the earth in the simplest way possible.

Each choice reflects values, beliefs, and the unique shape of a life.

The Role of Ritual After Death

They help families:

- pause long enough to feel
- gather in community
- speak the person's name
- remember who they were
- acknowledge the magnitude of the loss

Rituals also help the body catch up to what the heart already knows: someone beloved is gone.

Whether the ritual is ancient or newly invented, formal or improvised, it becomes part of the story the family carries forward.

What Families Remember

Years later, families rarely remember the logistics.
They remember the:

- music that made them cry
- story that made everyone laugh
- way sunlight fell across the room
- hands they held
- moment they felt the person's presence
- sense of community that carried them

They remember the love.

Funerals and celebrations of life are not about the body.
They are about the meaning of a life lived, the relationships formed, and the legacy left behind.

A Final Word for Families

The days after a death can feel surreal — a blur of decisions, paperwork, and emotion. But they also hold moments of profound beauty. Planning a farewell is an act of love. It is a way of saying:

- "This person mattered."

- "Their life touched ours."

- "We will carry them forward."

Whether the farewell is traditional or unconventional, religious or secular, simple or elaborate, what matters most is that it reflects the person's story.

A good death is shaped by values. A good farewell is shaped by love.

Chapter 27:

Grief and mourning

Grief is not a single emotion. It is a landscape — unpredictable, uneven, and deeply personal. It can include sorrow, anger, confusion, numbness, longing, and even moments of humor or relief. It does not move in a straight line, and it cannot be navigated quickly.

The Elizabeth Kübler-Ross stages of grief — denial, bargaining, anger, depression, acceptance — were never meant to be a rigid sequence. They are a vocabulary, not a map. People move back and forth among these emotions, sometimes within the same day, sometimes within the same hour. Grief is not a task to complete. It is a human response to love.

Loving deeply makes us vulnerable to profound sorrow. But that vulnerability is also evidence of the significance of the relationship. Grief honors the memory of those we love. It is the price of connection, and it reminds us that the joy of love is worth the inevitable sorrow that follows loss.

Yet grief can leave a person feeling unmoored — as if the world has shifted and nothing fits quite the same.

The Complexity of Grief

Grief is rarely simple because our deepest relationships are rarely simple. When the relationship had conflict, distance, dependence, or unresolved emotions, grief becomes layered. We mourn not only the person's absence but also the complexity of who they were to us.

Human relationships involve:

- love

- disappointment

- dependence

- conflict

- gratitude

- regret

When someone dies, the opportunity to address unfinished business disappears. This can leave the bereaved with lingering questions, unspoken apologies, and a sense of "what if." These feelings do not mean the relationship was flawed; they mean it was real.

Grieving often involves coming to terms with the imperfections of the deceased — and forgiving them for the pain they caused. Equally important is the need for **self-forgiveness**. Many people blame themselves for things left undone or unsaid. Working through these feelings is essential for healing, but it is not easy, especially when regret is strong.

Modern culture often tries to professionalize or pathologize grief — to treat it as something to be "fixed" or "overcome." While therapy and support can be invaluable, grief is not a disorder. It is a natural, communal, deeply human experience. It unfolds in its own time.

Mourning

If grief is the internal experience of loss, mourning is its external expression. Mourning gives shape to grief. It allows us to honor the person who died and to acknowledge the impact of their life within the community.

Mourning rituals — funerals, wakes, memorial services, celebrations of life — serve several purposes. They:

- provide structure during a time of emotional disorientation

- create a space for shared stories and collective remembrance

- reflect cultural, religious, and familial traditions

- help the bereaved begin to integrate the reality of the loss

Rituals do not erase grief. They give it a container. They mark the transition from presence to memory, helping the bereaved move from shock toward understanding.

Mourning is not a performance. It is a bridge — from the life that was shared to the life that must now continue.

Lessons Learned From the Death of a Loved One

Loss has a way of clarifying what matters. After the death of someone we love, we are reminded of:

- the importance of our connections to others

- what truly matters — relationships, presence, meaning

- the limits of medicine — what it can and cannot fix

- the value of preparation — emotional, practical, and spiritual

- the reality of impermanence — that life is finite

- the strengths and limits of caregivers — and the courage it takes to accompany someone to the end

- the necessity of facing our own mortality

These lessons are not abstract. They are lived. They shape how we love, how we plan, how we forgive, and how we choose to spend the time we have.

Grief changes us. Mourning helps us carry that change forward; and the love that remains becomes part of the story we continue to live.

Part VIII – THE RIGHT TO DIE

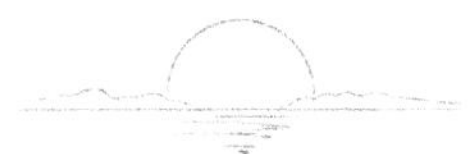

To die of old age is a death rare, extraordinary, and singular … a privilege rarely seen.
— Montaigne, Of Age, 1575 The Essays of Michel de Montaigne

Death is not extinguishing the light; it is only putting out the lamp because the dawn has come." — Rabindranath Tagore

Chapter 28:

The legal cases that started the Right to Die movement.

The modern right-to-die movement did not emerge from theory or philosophy. It emerged from families — ordinary people thrust into extraordinary circumstances — who found themselves fighting for the right to let a loved one die naturally. These landmark cases forced courts, clinicians, and the public to confront questions that medicine alone could not answer: What does it mean to be alive? Who decides when treatment becomes too much? And how do we honor a person's wishes when they can no longer speak for themselves?

The cases of Karen Ann Quinlan, Nancy Cruzan, Terri Schiavo, and Nancy Ellen Jobes reshaped American law and ethics. They also revealed the emotional cost of prolonged medical intervention and the moral weight placed on families who must decide when enough is enough.

Karen Ann Quinlan

The first state Supreme Court right-to-die case

On April 14, 1975, 21-year-old Karen Ann Quinlan collapsed at a party and slipped into a coma. She was placed on a ventilator and remained unresponsive. Her parents, believing she would not recover, asked that her endotracheal tube be removed so she could die naturally. The courts initially refused.

On March 31, 1976, the New Jersey Supreme Court issued a landmark ruling granting the Quinlan family the right to remove Karen's respirator. When the ventilator was discontinued on May 16, 1976, Karen continued to breathe on her own. She lived for nine more years, cared for in a nursing home, and died on June 11, 1985.

The Quinlan case prompted the passage of the **California Natural Death Act of 1976**, the first statute to acknowledge the legitimacy of private medical decisions. It firmly established the principle that individuals have the right to refuse or terminate medical treatment — a foundational concept in end-of-life law.

Nancy Cruzan

The first U.S. Supreme Court right-to-die case

In 1983, 25-year-old Nancy Cruzan suffered a car crash that left her in a persistent vegetative state. She required a feeding tube to survive. Her family sought to remove it, citing Nancy's earlier statements that she would not want to live in such a condition.

The case reached the U.S. Supreme Court in 1990. The Court ruled that competent adults have the constitutional right to refuse medical treatment — including artificial nutrition and hydration — and that states may require "clear and convincing evidence" of a patient's wishes.

After nearly eight years of litigation, the Cruzans met that standard. Nancy's feeding tube was removed, and she died twelve days later, on December 26, 1990.

The ruling affirmed that adults with decision-making capacity have the right to:

choose or refuse any medical intervention

decline artificial nutrition and hydration

create advance directives

appoint a surrogate decision-maker

It also affirmed that surrogates may decline treatment even if doing so will hasten death, as long as the intent is not to cause death but to honor the patient's wishes.

At Nancy's funeral, her father said, "I would prefer to have my daughter back and let someone else be this trailblazer." Six years later, overwhelmed by grief, he died by suicide.

Terri Schiavo

A national conflict over autonomy, family, and politics

In February 1990, 26-year-old Terri Schiavo collapsed at home, likely from a potassium imbalance related to bulimia. She suffered an anoxic brain injury and entered a persistent vegetative state. She could breathe on her own but required a PEG tube for nutrition.

Terri left no written instructions. Her husband, Michael, believed she would not want to live in this condition. Her parents believed she could improve with therapy. Every physician who examined her agreed she would never regain consciousness.

What followed was a **15-year legal battle** between Terri's husband and her parents — a conflict that drew national attention, political intervention, and public protest.

Key events included:

2000: A Florida judge ruled that Terri would refuse artificial feeding.

2001–2003: Her feeding tube was removed and reinserted multiple times due to legal challenges.

2003: The Florida Legislature passed "Terri's Law," allowing the governor to order the tube reinserted — nearly triggering a constitutional crisis.

2005: After another trial, the tube was removed for the final time. Terri died on March 31, 2005.

Her autopsy revealed profound brain atrophy — her brain weighed less than half of normal. No treatment could have reversed the damage.

The Schiavo case exposed emotional, ethical, and political turmoil that arises when a person's wishes are unknown.

Nancy Ellen Jobes

A case that expanded the right to withdraw artificial nutrition and hydration

In 1980, 24-year-old Nancy Ellen Jobes was pregnant when she was injured in a car crash. The fetus died and was surgically removed. During the procedure, Nancy suffered cardiac arrest due to an anesthesia complication, causing prolonged oxygen deprivation and irreversible brain damage. She entered a persistent vegetative state.

After five years with no improvement, her family sought permission to remove her feeding tube. A trial judge agreed but allowed the nursing home to refuse participation. The case reached the New Jersey Supreme Court, which upheld the family's right to withdraw artificial nutrition and hydration and removed the facility's discretion to decline.

Nancy was transferred to a hospital where the feeding tube was removed. She died on August 4, 1987.

Her case highlighted the tension between technological capability and humane care — and the moral conflict when institutions refuse to participate in withdrawing life-sustaining treatment even when the courts affirm the patient's rights.

The Right to Die: What These Cases Established

Over decades, the ethos of "keep the patient alive at all costs" has softened. Families and clinicians increasingly recognize that aggressive treatment is not always synonymous with good care.

These cases established that:

- individuals have the right to refuse medical treatment
- artificial nutrition and hydration are medical treatments, not moral obligations
- surrogates may decline treatment on a patient's behalf
- living wills and advance directives are essential
- states may require evidence of a patient's wishes
- clinicians are protected when they follow a patient's directives

Living Wills, however, have limitations. They cannot anticipate every scenario. They require interpretation. This is why **conversations** — about breathing tubes, feeding tubes, IV fluids, and the meaning of quality of life — are essential.

In North Carolina, the **Right to Natural Death Act** affirms a patient's right to decline life-prolonging measures and allows individuals to express the deeper meaning behind their choices. It protects clinicians who honor those directives and prohibits active euthanasia.

Who Decides What "Quality of Life" Means?

Quality of life is deeply personal. Many people with profound disabilities describe their lives as meaningful and full. Their voices remind us that quality cannot be reduced to physical function alone.

But the slope becomes slippery when others make those judgments on someone else's behalf. For instance, if an adult child wants a parent designated DNR, what is motivating that decision?

- love

- fear

- exhaustion

- financial strain

- misunderstanding

These questions matter.

At the same time, keeping someone "nominally alive" through technology raises its own moral weight. Some groups insist that life must be preserved at all costs. They are entitled to that belief — for their own lives. But many have never witnessed the contracted, dependent existence of someone living in a nursing home with no hope of recovery.

The New Jersey Supreme Court recognized this in the Jobes case:

- **The people best equipped to decide are those who know the patient most intimately.**

Yet larger forces — institutions, legislators, political movements — increasingly shape how we die.

Ultimately, the central question becomes:
What is the goal?

- *prolonging biological life*

- *preserving dignity*

- *honoring the person's values*

These goals are not always aligned.

A Personal Reflection on the Right to Die

For me, the right to die is not abstract. My mother made her wishes clear: no resuscitation, no machines, no aggressive attempts to prolong a life that was naturally ending. Hospice helped us care for her at home. She died in her own bed, surrounded by familiarity and dignity.

I have done everything within my power to make my own wishes known — a living will, a primary and secondary healthcare proxy, conversations with my family. And yet I still wonder: will the system override me anyway?

If I were lying in a bed, partially conscious, kept alive by tubes against my stated wishes, and had even one clear thought, I would be furious.

I hope my children never see me in the full deterioration of disease. I want them to remember the thousand moments of joy we shared — not the decline.

When Technology Prolongs Dying

Over the years, I have cared for thousands of patients whose bodies dwindled until nothing remained but the machinery keeping them alive. One patient had been on our unit for weeks. His son said, "I can't choose to remove the tubes. God must choose."

But if one believes in an all-powerful God who allowed the heart attack — hadn't God already chosen? As we perform the surgeries, insert the tubes, and do all the endless interventions, aren't we the ones refusing to let that choice unfold?

Every day before the son arrived, I bathed his father, changed dressings, combed his hair, and arranged his sheets. What the son didn't see was the reality beneath the tidy surface, the:

- infected stump from an amputation

- yellowing skin of liver failure

- profound confusion

- suffering

We call this "extraordinary care," but often it feels like unnatural care.

If he survived long enough to reach a nursing home, he would likely:

- develop contractures

- become incontinent

- suffer skin breakdown

- endure bedsores

- stare at the walls for years

Tube feedings would continue and life could continue — indefinitely. Is that a natural death?

Families visit, but their lives continue. The patient remains suspended — alive in the biological sense, but gone in every meaningful way.

The emotional, physical, and financial cost is staggering.

PART IX — CONCLUSION

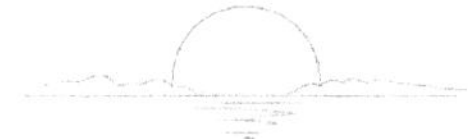

Twenty years from now you will be more disappointed by the things that you didn't do than by the ones you did do. So, throw off the bowlines. Sail away from the safe harbor. Catch the trade winds in your sails. Explore. Dream. Discover.
— H. Jackson Brown Jr.

To live is the rarest thing in the world. Most people exist, that is all.
— Oscar Wilde

You are a droplet of consciousness that separated from the ocean to explore a body, a name, and a story. But a droplet doesn't stop being water just because it's a droplet. Death is simply the moment the droplet returns to the sea. This isn't a tragedy; it is a completion. You are returning to the field of wholeness.
— Mitchell Roth

Chapter 29

My Reality

I've brushed up against the possibility of dying more than once. I walked away from two totaled cars, one of which left me with a basilar skull fracture and lower spinal disc damage. Then, in my early twenties, I had a fallopian tube tumor removed in August. Just a few months later, in October, I found a lump in my neck. My doctors feared it might be metastasis from the tumor they had removed. The ENT specialist didn't soften his words: "It could be lymphoma. If it's metastatic disease, you may have about six months. We won't know until we take it out."

I had to wait several weeks for surgery — weeks that felt like their own strange, suspended world. I moved back home with my parents. Watching my mother worry was its own kind of heartbreak. She didn't say much, but she stayed in her bedroom with the door closed; when she came out, her eyes were swollen. Anxiety and sadness filled the house.

And yet, during those weeks, everything around me sharpened. The world looked brighter, more vivid, more fragile. Things I used to worry about suddenly felt trivial. What mattered were sunsets, balloons, my friends, cats, peanut butter, my family — all the small, ordinary miracles I had taken for granted.

At twenty-one, four days before Christmas, I went into surgery. The plan was simple on paper but terrifying in reality: if the mass was cancer, the surgeons would immediately perform a radical neck dissection. That meant removing part of my jaw, the main neck muscle that turns the head, the internal jugular vein, a crucial spinal nerve, and all the lymph nodes and surrounding tissue. I might wake up disfigured. I might wake up unable to move my head. I might wake up with only an incision. I hadn't even been in love yet. And I was only twenty-one.

In the end, the lump wasn't cancer. The fallopian tube tumor wasn't cancer either — the biopsy had been right all along. The lump was "just" an infected lymph node that had pushed my submandibular salivary gland outward. I did lose movement on the left side of my face for a while, and only about half of it ever returned, but I was alive — and mostly intact. I was deeply, overwhelmingly grateful.

The experience changed me in ways I still can't fully articulate. Even after I returned to my college life, the awareness stayed with me.

It taught me to think about what truly matters. I still get angry, sad, or overwhelmed by life's problems — big and small — and I get so frustrated with myself when I forget what I know. But underneath all of that, I carry a deeper awareness of how sweet life really is. When I pause, even for a moment, gratitude rises. I am thankful for this life, every bit of it.

Reflections on Living While We Can

When you start to understand that each day lived isn't an extra day added, but one fewer remaining, you begin to see the things that really matter.

These are the truths that have shaped how I try to live with intention daily:

- ### Overlooked Moments

Most of us spend more time waiting than living. We wait for the weekend, the next holiday, the next milestone. But life happens in the ordinary moments we overlook. The end of life makes this unmistakably clear.

- ### This moment is the only one we truly have

Life unfolds in the breath you're taking now, in the conversation you're having today, in the small choices you make without fanfare. The present is the only place where anything real occurs.

- ### A lifetime is shorter than it appears from the middle

We imagine decades ahead — until life teaches us otherwise. Not everyone gets eighty years. Not everyone gets tomorrow. If something matters, begin. If someone matters, tell them.

- ### What we invest in now shapes the life we leave behind

Meaning is built slowly — through relationships, purpose, craft, clarity. Preparing for death means asking: *What am I building with the time I have left?*

- ### Putting things off is its own burden

Procrastination delays more than tasks; it delays peace. Even one small step toward what we've avoided lightens tomorrow. One person said that if life didn't have an expiration date, nothing would ever get done.

• Failure is part of being human

No one reaches the end of life without mistakes. These experiences shape us; they do not diminish us.

• The relationship we have with ourselves sets the tone for everything else

Mortality strips away the need to impress. What remains is honesty — about what we want, what we fear, and who we are.

• People reveal themselves through what they do, not what they promise

As life narrows, clarity sharpens. We see who shows up, who keeps their word, who brings calm instead of chaos.

• Kindness is one of the few things that endures

People rarely remember accomplishments near the end of life. They remember how you made them feel.

• Struggle is woven into every meaningful life

Difficulty is universal. The ability to keep going, to adapt, to love despite loss — that is the quiet strength that carries people throughout their life and their final days.

• Preparing for death is ultimately about living with intention now

A life lived with intention naturally leads to a death met with readiness. When we tend to what matters, the end becomes less frightening — not because it changes, but because we do.

And Finally

I once sat with a hospice patient who asked me a question I wasn't prepared for. She had been given a terminal diagnosis — about a year to live — yet she still felt well. She looked at me and asked:

"I don't know how much time I really have… should I travel? Should I go see all my friends and family across the country?"

At the time, I stumbled through an answer about doing whatever she truly wanted. But her question stayed with me. Over the years, I've realized a deeper truth. Every one of us has a terminal diagnosis; not one pronounced by a physician. We are all going to die.

Some of us are forced to confront that reality because illness interrupts our lives. The rest of us move through our days as if the end is theoretical, far away, or optional — pretending we have unlimited time.

Whether our death comes today or decades from now, the fact remains: our time is finite. And with that awareness, isn't it remarkable that we can choose to live with purpose — consciously, every day — to shape a life filled with intention, joy, and meaning, instead of waiting for a diagnosis to remind us?

About the Author

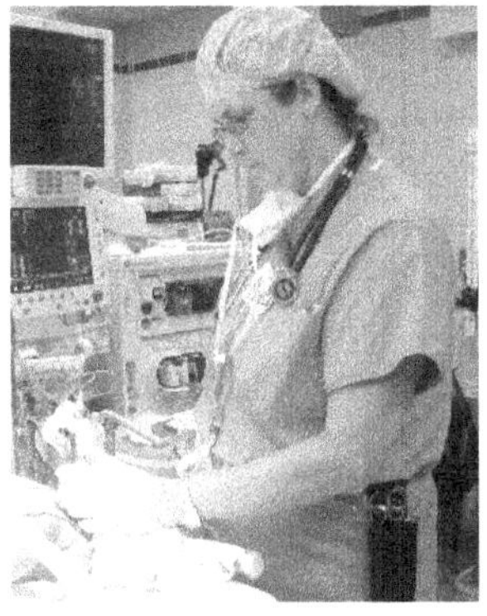

Lynn Fitzgerald Macksey, RN, MSN, CRNA, has spent more than four decades in the intimate spaces where medicine meets meaning. She began her career as an EMT and LPN, earned her BSN in 1985, and went on to work in cardiac and critical care units, open-heart ICUs, neuro-trauma services, surgical recovery, and hospice care. She has cared for patients in their first minutes of life and their last — in intensive care, trauma bays, and quiet hospice bedrooms where families whisper their goodbyes.

After twenty-three years of bedside critical care nursing, Lynn attended the University of Pittsburgh to become a Certified Registered Nurse Anesthetist. Her clinical path in anesthesia took her from Pennsylvania to North Carolina, where she practiced for twenty-three years — the last decade at the University of North Carolina at Chapel Hill. She has taught and precepted nurse anesthesia students and anesthesiology residents, lectured internationally, and authored multiple anesthesia textbooks and case reports. Her work reflects a rare combination of technical mastery and emotional clarity.

But Lynn's understanding of mortality is not only professional. She has faced her own brushes with death, cared for both her father and mother through their final months, and witnessed thousands of families navigating the fragile space between hope and acceptance. These experiences deepened her belief that preparing for death is ultimately about living with intention — noticing the small miracles, tending to what matters, and allowing love to guide the choices we make.

Lynn now lives in North Carolina with her husband of forty-one years, Keith, and their pets, grateful every day for the sweetness of ordinary life.

- **Advance Directive**: a legal document stating a person's wishes for medical care if they cannot speak for themselves.

- **Analgesia**: relief from pain.

- **Anticipatory grief**: grief experienced before a loss occurs.

- **Apnea**: pause in breathing, most often temporary.

- **Artificial nutrition & hydration**: tube feeding or IV nutrition when a person cannot eat or drink.

- **Brain death**: irreversible loss of all brain function; legally recognized as death.

- **Cardiac arrest**: sudden stopping of the heart.

- **Comfort care**: care focused on relief of symptoms rather than cure.

- **Cardiac catheterization**: a medical procedure in which a flexible tube called a catheter is inserted into a blood vessel in the wrist or groin and guided to the heart to diagnose and sometimes treat a heart condition.

- **CPR (Cardiopulmonary Resuscitation)**: emergency procedure to restart breathing or heartbeat.

- **Critical Care**: specialized care for life-threatening conditions.

- **Denial of death**: a psychological response in which a person avoids, minimizes, or rejects the reality of death to protect a person emotionally.

- **Defibrillation**: the delivery of a controlled electric shock to the heart (through the chest wall) to stop a life-threatening arrhythmia in hopes that the heart's normal rhythm will restart.

- **Dialysis**: a medical treatment that removes waste products, toxins, and excess fluid from the blood when the kidneys are no longer able to do so effectively.

- **DNR (Do Not Resuscitate)**: a medical order instructing providers not to perform CPR.

- **DNI (Do Not Intubate)**: a medical order to not place a breathing tube if a person stops breathing.

- **Dyspnea**: difficulty or discomfort in breathing.
- **EMS**: Emergency Medical Services (EMS) typically includes paramedics, emergency medical technicians (EMT), ambulance crews, first responders (firefighters, police officers, trained volunteers).
- **End-of-Life Care**: support and treatment during the final phase of life.
- **Ethics, medical**: principles and values that guide how healthcare professionals make decisions, treat patients, and balance competing needs. These values are based on being fair, compassionate, respectful and aligned with a patient's rights and dignity.
- **Extubation**: removal of a breathing tube.
- **Family meeting**: a structured discussion between clinicians and family about goals of care.
- **Feeding tube**: a tube that provides nutrition, fluids, or medications to a person who cannot eat or swallow safely on their own. It delivers this directly into the stomach or intestines, or into the nose and down in the esophagus.
- **Foley catheter**: a catheter that has been placed into the bladder to drain urine.
- **Full Code**: a default to perform all life-saving measures, including CPR and intubation.
- **Goals of care**: the patient's priorities for treatment, comfort, and quality of life.
- **Hospice**: care for people with a life expectancy of six months or less, focused on comfort.
- **Hospitalist**: a doctor who cares for patients only while they are in the hospital.
- **ICU (Intensive Care Unit)**: Hospital unit for critically ill patients needing close monitoring.
- **Informed consent**: process in which a patient is given clear, understandable information about a medical test, treatment, or procedure, and then voluntarily agrees to it. It is a legal/ethical requirement.
- **Intensivist**: a doctor who specializes in critical care medicine, working primarily in the intensive care unit. They are experts in managing life-threatening conditions.

- **Intra-aortic balloon pump**: a short-term mechanical device placed in the aorta to support a failing heart by improving blood flow to the coronary arteries. It is inserted into a leg artery.

- **Intravenous (IV) infusion**: delivery of fluids or medications directly into a vein.

- **Intubation**: placement of a tube into the airway to assist breathing.

- **Invasive procedure**: medical intervention that enters the body, either by breaking the skin or by inserting instruments into natural body openings. They range from minor to highly complex.

- **Life-sustaining treatment**: interventions that prolong life (ventilators, dialysis, CPR).

- **Living Will**: a type of advance directive describing desired medical treatments.

- **Lung Protective Ventilation**: a ventilator strategy to reduce lung injury.

- **Mechanical ventilation**: machine-assisted breathing.

- **Medical interventions**: actions, treatments, or procedures performed by healthcare professionals to diagnose, prevent, manage, or treat health conditions.

- **Mottling**: blotchy skin pattern often seen near the end of life.

- **Morphine drip**: continuous infusion of morphine for pain or breathlessness.

- **NIV (Non-Invasive Ventilation)**: breathing support using a mask instead of a tube.

- **Organ donation**: giving organs after death for transplantation.

- **Palliative care**: specialized care focused on quality of life and symptom relief at any stage of illness.

- **Palliative sedation**: medication used to reduce severe, refractory suffering at end of life.

- **Pneumonia**: an infection of the lungs that causes the alveoli (air sacs) to fill with fluid, pus, or inflammatory cells.

- **Post-mortem care**: care provided after death to prepare the body.

- **Prognosis**: expected course or outcome of a disease.

- **Proxy**: a person who is legally or formally authorized to make decisions on someone else's behalf when that person cannot speak or act for themselves.

- **Pulse oximetry**: a device that measures oxygen saturation.

- **Rapid Response Team**: clinicians who respond to sudden patient deterioration.

- **Respiratory failure**: inability of the lungs to provide adequate oxygen or remove carbon dioxide.

- **Respite care**: temporary relief for caregivers.

- **Sepsis**: life-threatening condition that begins with an infection but moves to an extreme response leading to organ dysfunction.

- **Symptom management**: treatment of pain, nausea, anxiety, breathlessness, etc.

- **Terminal extubation**: removal of a breathing tube when the goal is comfort at end of life.

- **Tracheostomy**: a medical procedure in which a surgeon creates an opening in the front of the neck directly into the trachea (windpipe) to help a person breath when they need long-term breathing support.

- **Transition of care**: moving from curative treatment to comfort-focused care.

- **Unresponsive**: not reacting to voice or touch.

- **Vasopressors**: intravenous medications that raise blood pressure by constricting blood vessels and sometimes help the heart pump more effectively. Given when the blood pressure is dangerously low.

- **Ventilator**: machine that supports or replaces breathing.

- **Ventilator withdrawal**: stopping mechanical ventilation when aligned with goals of care.

- **Vital signs**: measures of basic body function (heart rate, blood pressure, temperature, breathing rate).

- **Withholding treatment**: not starting a treatment that is unlikely to help or not desired.

- **Withdrawal of care**: stopping treatments that no longer align with patient goals.